Maria Tereza S.L.R. Borges
Geraldo Bezerra da Silva Junior
Zélia Maria S.A. Santos

Adherence to treatment for systemic arterial hypertension

Maria Tereza S.L.R. Borges
Geraldo Bezerra da Silva Junior
Zélia Maria S.A. Santos

Adherence to treatment for systemic arterial hypertension

Construction and validation of an assessment technology

ScienciaScripts

Imprint

Cover image: www.ingimage.com

This book is a translation from the original published under ISBN 978-613-9-61899-6.

Publisher:
Sciencia Scripts
is a trademark of
Dodo Books Indian Ocean Ltd. and OmniScriptum S.R.L publishing group

120 High Road, East Finchley, London, N2 9ED, United Kingdom
Str. Armeneasca 28/1, office 1, Chisinau MD-2012, Republic of Moldova, Europe
Printed at: see last page
ISBN: 978-620-7-70708-9

SUMMARY

MARIA TEREZA SA LEITAO RAMOS BORGES

Master's Degree in Collective Health from the University of Fortaleza-UNIFOR. Graduated in Medicine from the Federal University of Cearà (1983). Medical residency in Internal Medicine and Cardiology. She is currently an intensive care physician at the Dr. José Frota Institute - Fortaleza City Hall, Intensive care physician - Coronary Unit - Messejana Hospital - Preceptor of the Cardiology Residency - Messejana Hospital - Specialist in cardiology by the Brazilian Society of Cardiology (SBC).Specialist in Intensive Care from the Brazilian Intensive Care Medical Association (AMIB) - Postgraduate course in Critical Patient Care Management - Sirio Libanês Hospital -SP-Sao Paulo - Medical Consultancy - working mainly on the following subjects: cardiology, arterial hypertension-medical clinic and intensive care-Researcher at NUESPHA-UNIFOR (Nùcleo de Ensino e Pesquisa em Hipertensao Arterial).

ZÉLIA MARIA DE SOUSA ARAÙJO SANTOS

Graduated in Nursing from the Federal University of Cearà (UFC) in 1980, and in Administration from the State University of Cearà (UECE) in 1985. Specialist in Arterial Hypertension by the Brazilian Society of Hypertension (SBH) since 2001. Master's and Doctorate in Nursing from the UFC in 1998 and 2001, respectively. Post-Doctorate in Collective Health from the Collective Health Institute (ISC) of the Federal University of Bahia (UFBA) in 2009. Full Professor of the Nursing Course, the Postgraduate Program in Collective Health (PPGSC) and the Professional Master's Degree - Technology and Innovation in Nursing (MPTIE) at the University of Fortaleza (UNIFOR). Leader of the Study, Research and Extension Center for the Promotion of the Health of People with Arterial Hypertension (NUESPHA), linked to the Research Line - Policies and Practices in the Promotion of Health of the Research Group - Policies and Practices in the Promotion of Health/CNPq.

GERALDO BEZERRA DA SILVA JUNIOR

Graduated in Medicine from the Federal University of Cearà; Residency in Clinical Medicine at the César Cals General Hospital, of the Health Department of the State of Cearà; Residency in Nephrology at the Walter Cantidio University Hospital of the Federal University of Cearà; Master's and Doctorate in Medical Sciences from the Federal University of Cearà; Post-Doctorate in Collective Health and Epidemiology from the Federal University of Bahia. He is currently Adjunct Professor of Medicine and of the Postgraduate Programs in Collective Health and Medical Sciences at the University of Fortaleza and Physician at the Federal Institute of Education, Science and Technology of Cearà. He has experience in the field of Medicine, working mainly in the areas of Clinical Medicine and Nephrology. He also conducts research in the areas of Internal Medicine,

Nephrology, Tropical Medicine, Public Health and Medical Education, with an emphasis on kidney diseases. Member of the Brazilian Society of Nephrology and the International Society of Nephrology.

PRESENTATION

Hypertension: A public health problem and a global challenge

Systemic Arterial Hypertension (SAH) is considered by the World Health Organization to be the leading cause of death worldwide, with figures close to nine million people a year (WHO, 2013). It affects approximately one in four adults and reduces life expectancy by between 10 and 15 years.

It is estimated that by the year 2020, deaths from cardiovascular diseases will increase by 15 to 20%, and by the year 2030, chronic non-communicable diseases will be responsible for 75% of deaths worldwide (WHO, 2011), i.e. it is estimated that by the year 2030 around 23.6 million people will die from cardiovascular diseases, and it is predicted that they will continue to be the main cause of death globally.

One of the most important factors explaining the impact of the burden of disease and mortality from cardiovascular diseases is the demographic transition. There are more people on the planet today, with a relative increase in life expectancy at birth, which will allow more of them to grow old enough to develop cardiovascular diseases. Considering the predicted trends in world population ageing, it is estimated that around 10% of the current world population aged over 60 will increase to 16.6% by 2030 and 21.4% by 2050 (ABEGUNDE *et al,* 2007).

The profound change in demographic trends requires priority attention. These changes have an impact on social organization, values and individual behavioural norms - examples include risk factors such as metabolic disorders, eating disorders, abdominal obesity, consumption of illicit substances and changes in healthy lifestyles - and on families; they also have implications for the socio-economic field and for education, health and social security systems, among others (ABEGUNDE *et al,* 2007; MONCAYO, 2011). Finally, other related factors that cannot be overlooked are those associated with poverty and inequality in the distribution of wealth between social groups, as well as access to healthy and innocuous food, food safety, cultural differences and access to good quality health services.

The fight against cardiovascular disease requires a coordinated multisectoral response. Health policies, research strategies and health systems around the world, especially in developing countries, must be adapted and strengthened to deal with diseases that tend to develop later in life. Strategies must be developed that target individuals and populations. There are several randomized controlled studies of education conducted by nurses to change behaviour in primary care. These studies show that the groups of patients who underwent intervention achieved greater changes in habits, and these changes were maintained over 4 to 12 months of follow-up (Wood et al, 2008). To this end, comprehensive action at national, regional and global level is urgent and mandatory in order to guarantee effective measures to prevent mortality, sequelae and mitigate the progression of cardiovascular disease.

As with other non-communicable diseases, awareness-raising helps with early detection, and self-monitoring helps to ensure compliance with pharmacological treatment, healthy behaviors and better control of the disease.

High-income Western countries on the old continent have begun to reduce hypertension in their populations through rigorous public policies, such as reducing salt in processed foods and making diagnosis and treatment services for hypertension and other risk factors widely available. Numerous examples can be mentioned of joint, intersectoral actions that effectively tackle hypertension risk factors. A good example of good public policy practices for hypertension control is Portugal, one of the first European Union countries to draw up a national law in 2009 to limit the maximum amount of salt in bread (1.4 grams of salt per 100 grams of the final product or 0.55 grams of sodium), since various studies suggest that bread contributes high levels to the population's total intake. In contrast, in many developing countries the number of people suffering heart attacks and cerebrovascular accidents caused by undiagnosed and uncontrolled risk factors, such as hypertension, is increasing.

In this book, the authors review the state of the art and information on hypertension, its prevalence, the level of knowledge, the extent of its control and treatment, in order to develop and apply policies aimed at reducing mortality and the loss of years due to disability caused by hypertension. Studies are presented on the application of technology to assess hypertensive patients' adherence to treatment, the results of multidisciplinary intervention, its interaction with other cardiovascular risk factors and some aspects of the updated international guidelines for its management. Prevention and control of hypertension are the cornerstones of a global public health policy in the 21st century.

José Manuel Peixoto Caldas

Physician and Sociologist. Institute of Public Health, University of Porto, Portugal. Full Professor at the Federal University of Paraiba, Brazil. Coordinator of the Global Public Health Program.

E-mail: jcaldas@fpce.up.pt, jcaldas@ccs.ufpb.br

References

World Health Organization. General information on hypertension in the world. Geneva: Switzerland, 2013.

World Health Organization. Global status report on non communicable diseases. Geneva: Switzerland, 2011. **World Health Organization.** New HWO report. April 27, Geneva: Switzerland, 2011.

Abegunde DO, Mathers CD, Adam T, Ortegon M, Strong K. The burden and costs of chronic diseases in low-income and middle-income countries. Lancet. 2007; 370:1929-38

Moncayo A. New dimensions of public health. En: Malagón-Londono G, Moncayo-Medina A, editors. Public Health.

Perspectives. Second edition. Bogotà: Editorial Médica Panamericana; 2011. p. 26-44.

Wood D, Kotseva K, Connolly S, et al. EUROACTION Study Group.Nurse- coordinated multidisciplinary, family-based cardiovascular disease prevention program (EUROACTION) for patients with coronary heart disease and asymptomatic individuals at high risk of cardiovascular disease: a paired,cluster-randomized controlled trial. Lancet. 2008 Jun 14; 371(9629):1999-2012.

1. INTRODUCTION

Systemic arterial hypertension (SAH) is a multifactorial clinical condition characterized by high and sustained levels of blood pressure (BP) ≥140 and/or 90 mmHg. It affects a large part of the world's population and, when not treated properly, brings major and serious complications to its sufferers. Some of these changes are due to non-adherence to treatment or inadequate treatment. It is often associated with metabolic, functional and/or structural alterations in target organs. It is aggravated by the presence of other risk factors (RF), such as abdominal obesity, dyslipidemia, glucose intolerance and diabetes mellitus (DM). It is independently associated with cardiovascular (CV) events such as sudden death, stroke, heart failure, acute myocardial infarction, peripheral arterial disease and chronic kidney disease, both fatal and non-fatal. Complications occur due to impairment of target organs (kidneys, heart, brain and blood vessels) (DBHA, 2016; VASAN, 2002). It is aggravated by the presence of other risk factors (RF), such as dyslipidemia, abdominal obesity, glucose intolerance and *diabetes mellitus (*DM). There is an independent association with events such as sudden death, stroke, acute myocardial infarction (AMI), heart failure (HF), peripheral arterial disease (PAD) and chronic kidney disease (CKD) (DBHA, 2016).

In developed countries, non-adherence to treatment for chronic diseases hovers around 50%, and is probably higher in developing countries. Among these diseases, hypertension is asymptomatic and has an impact on the user upon diagnosis, especially with regard to the use of medication and lifestyle changes (WHO, 2003).

In Brazil, AH affects 32.5% (36 million) of adults and more than 60% of the elderly, leading to 50% of deaths from cardiovascular disease (CVD).7 Together with DM, its complications (heart, kidney and stroke) have a high impact on the loss of labor productivity and family income, estimated at US$ 4.18 billion between 2006 and 2015.

There is a direct, linear association between ageing and the prevalence of SAH, related to the increase in life expectancy of the Brazilian population, currently 74.9 years, and the increase in the population of elderly people ≥ 60 years in the last decade (2000 to 2010), from 6.7% to 10.8%. In Brazil, the average diagnosis of hypertension in the 27 Brazilian state capitals studied was 22.7%, and was higher in women (25.4%) than in men (19.5%). The frequency of diagnosis increased with age for both sexes, more markedly for women, reaching 5.9% between the ages of 18-24 and more than 50% in the 50+ age group. In Fortaleza, the percentage of diagnoses was 17.3%, 11.2% in males and 19.8% in females. Chronic non-communicable diseases (CNCDs) are responsible for 72% of the causes of death in Brazil (BRASIL, 2009; BRASIL, 2012).

According to the World Health Organization (WHO) (2012), one in three adults aged 25 or over suffers from SAH. In Brazil, data from the Ministry of Health (MS) in a survey of 54,000 Brazilians in 2011 revealed that SAH affects 22.7% of the adult population (BRASIL, 2013).

Recent data reveal a prevalence of 32.5% (36 million) of adults, of which around 60% are elderly, contributing to 50% of deaths from cardiovascular diseases in Brazil (DBHA, 2016).

The prevalence of SAH has risen in recent years as a result of increased life expectancy, obesity and diabetes mellitus. On the other hand, the time to onset of this condition has declined due to preventive and health-promoting efforts aimed at individuals with pre-HAS (CEARA, 2013).

It has been observed that there is low adherence of hypertensive users to treatment, and this contributes to the development of acute, acute chronic and chronic complications, such as stroke, hypertensive encephalopathy, acute pulmonary edema, acute aortic dissection, acute coronary syndromes and other complications (YUSUF, 2004).

The essence is to provide society with health promotion, prevention and cure services, through the interdisciplinary work of multi-professional health teams and to promote training in universities for these professionals who deal with people with hypertension, with the aim of practicing greater guidance and management of this pathology, contributing to greater adherence to treatment in individuals with this pathology, which contributes to increased costs and risks of cardiovascular events as a result of inadequate BP control (BUS, 2003; MACHADO, 2012).

The individual's participation should be encouraged, giving them responsibility for the success of their treatment, with an active attitude of participation and complicity. Ask them what their participation should be and make them aware of the importance of their commitment to their treatment (CANESQUI, 2007). Support from the multidisciplinary health team is essential, in a relationship of working together voluntarily, both for pharmacological treatment and for developing health behaviors.

Controlling blood pressure (BP) is directly linked to reducing the problems caused by hypertension. It is therefore of great importance that patients with high BP are treated so that they can enjoy the benefits of anti-hypertensive treatment (NOBRE, 2010).

Problems with absent signs and symptoms, such as SAH, require the participation of the health team in order to make the user aware of the seriousness of the treatment and its benefits through preventive and health promotion activities (JARDIM, 2007).

Adherence to treatment is a subject that has been much studied, as it is very comprehensive, complex and a public health issue. Facilitating adherence to treatment means preventing complications and problems and providing quality of life (ALHALAIQA, 2012).

Assessing adherence to treatment for hypertension is important for monitoring hypertensive patients, and its multidimensionality must be taken into account, i.e. the various factors that determine adherence - biological and sociocultural characteristics, experiences with the disease and treatment, the relationship between the health team and the user, family participation, and access to the health system (WHO, 2003).

It should be emphasized that the need to develop technology to assess adherence to treatment for a chronic disease with a high prevalence, morbidity and mortality rate is one of the Ministry of Health's research priorities (ALMEIDA, 2008). In this context, SAH is mentioned because it is a major problem for public health.

The treatment of hypertension consists of lifestyle changes and the adoption of healthy habits through hygiene measures and drug treatment when indicated (SANTOS, 2012). The technology used to assess adherence to SAH treatment should include both non-pharmacological (or basic) and pharmacological treatment. Non-pharmacological (or basic) treatment involves the adoption of a healthy lifestyle - healthy eating, regular physical exercise, abstention from addictions, adequate consumption of alcoholic and caffeine-containing beverages, and stress management; and pharmacological treatment includes the adequate and regular use of antihypertensive medication.

This study was chosen because of the results of literature reviews on the focus and effectiveness of the available instruments used to assess adherence to treatment. A systematic review carried out by Leandro (2013) found that the instruments available exclusively assess adherence to drug treatment. This is a major gap, since this treatment modality is associated, according to risk stratification, when basic treatment alone does not control BP. Therefore, the instrument should assess adherence to both treatment modalities. Also based on this study, in relation to effectiveness, the *Morisky Green* instrument stood out. Therefore, given the problem of adherence to treatment and the need for an instrument that evaluates the two modalities of treatment for hypertension - basic and medication, this study consisted of the construction and validation of a technology for evaluating hypertensive users' adherence to treatment, regardless of the modalities indicated.

2. ARTERIAL HYPERTENSION - a public health problem

Concept and epidemiology. The prevalence of SAH is around 30-45% of the general population and increases with age. It is defined as systemic blood pressure (SBP) greater than or equal to 140 mmHg and diastolic blood pressure (DBP) greater than or equal to 90 mmHg. This classification is valid for young people, middle-aged adults and the elderly (ESH, 2013).

The prevalence of uncontrolled BP ranges from 50-59%. It is estimated that only a third of people regularly followed up in health services have their BP maintained at desirable levels. It is a chronic multifactorial disease, often detected late due to its slow and silent evolution (DBHA, 2016).

SAH has an independent and continuous relationship with the incidence of stroke, acute myocardial infarction (AMI), sudden death, heart failure, peripheral arterial disease and end-stage renal disease, which occurs in all ages and ethnicities (ESH, 2013).

Classification. BP levels are classified in mmHg as normal (SBP ≤120mmHg and DBP≤80mmHg), pre-hypertension (SBP of 121-139mmHg and/or DBP of 8189mmHg), stage 1 hypertension (SBP of 140-159mmHg and/or DBP of 90-99mmHg), stage 2 hypertension (SBP of 160-179mmHg and/or DBP of 100-109mmHg), grade 3 hypertension (SBP>= 180 and/or DBP >=110) and isolated systemic hypertension (SBP>=140 and DBP< 90). The category is defined by the highest level of systolic or diastolic BP. Isolated systolic hypertension can be grade 1, 2 or 3 according to the SBP values observed (DBHA, 2016).

ISH is common in healthy young men under 30 and may be associated with normal central pressure. Treatment would not have significant benefits, and the adoption of non-drug measures, with LOA monitoring, is recommended. The treatment of ISH should begin immediately with pharmacological therapy if the CV risk is high. In the event of a rise in DBP, the same treatment criteria are adopted as for the general population.

It is recommended to start pharmacological antihypertensive therapy in the elderly from SBP levels ≥ 140 mmHg, as long as it is well tolerated and the individual's general condition is assessed. In the very elderly, i.e. those aged ≥ 80 years, the threshold for starting pharmacological therapy increases to a SBP ≥ 160 mmHg.

It can be classified as primary or secondary. It is primary when it has no reversible cause, and secondary when it has a specific, potentially reversible cause and occurs in a small proportion of adult patients. However, in view of the high prevalence of hypertension, secondary forms can affect millions of people worldwide and if diagnosed and treated the patient can be cured or control their BP and reduce cardiovascular risks. All hypertensive people should be evaluated for secondary hypertension. It can be indicated by a severe rise in BP, difficulty in controlling BP and the presence of target organ damage, disproportionate to the time of diagnosis of the disease. Common causes of secondary SAH are: renal parenchymal disease, renal artery stenosis, primary aldosteronism and the uncommon ones: pheochromocytoma and *Cushing's syndrome* (ESH, 2013).

Secondary SAH has a prevalence of 3-5%. Treating its cause can cure or improve BP control (DBHA, 2016).

Resistant hypertension is office BP that is not controlled with the use of three or more antihypertensive drugs in adequate doses, including a diuretic, or with the use of four or more pressure-controlling drugs. It has a prevalence of 12% of the hypertensive population.

Refractory hypertension is uncontrolled BP when taking five or more antihypertensive drugs. Its prevalence is 3.6% of resistant hypertensive patients.

Clinical manifestations and diagnosis. As this is an asymptomatic syndrome that is slow to develop, a careful clinical assessment should be carried out on an individual with presumed hypertension. Initially, SAH should be confirmed, target organ damage should be identified, CVRF should be identified, the presence of comorbidities should be assessed, followed by overall cardiovascular risk. A probable cause of secondary SAH should also be identified (DBHA, 2016). Diagnosis includes BP measurement and clinical history, including family history, physical examination and laboratory investigations (ESH, 2013).

Due to the difficulty in finding mercury sphygmomanometers, auscultatory and semi-automatic sphygmomanometers are used to measure BP, which must be automatically calibrated in technical laboratories. Mercury column sphygmomanometers are ideal for these measurements as they are more accurate. Aneroid-type devices, when used, should be periodically tested and properly calibrated. BP should be checked in both arms. The size of the cuff should be adapted to the circumference of the patient's arm. If there is a significant difference between the two arms (>1 OmmHg), this may be associated with increased cardiovascular risk and the arm with the higher value should be used. Check weight, height, BMI, heart rate (HR), abdominal circumference and signs of secondary hypertension. In elderly and diabetic patients, BP should be assessed about 3 minutes in the orthostatic position to assess postural hypotension (defined as a reduction of >20mmHg in SBP and > IOmmHg in DBP), which is related to higher mortality and cardiovascular events (ESH, 2013) (DBHA, 2016).

The clinical history should include the period of the first diagnosis of hypertension, the BP values recorded, the use of medication and attention to signs of secondary hypertension. Women should be asked about hypertension during pregnancy and hormone replacement. Assess the presence of diabetes, clinical signs or history of heart failure, coronary artery disease, heart valve disease, palpitations, syncopal episodes, neurological disorders, stroke, transient ischemic attack (TIA), kidney disease, nicotine use, presence of dyslipidemia. An early family history of SAH and/or cardiovascular disease (CVD) should also be assessed (ESH, 2013).

Laboratory investigations (ESH/ESC, 2013). The purpose of laboratory investigations is to identify the presence of risk factors (RF), target organ damage and secondary SAH.

Routine tests. Hematocrit and hemoglobin, fasting glucose, total cholesterol and fractions, triglycerides, serum potassium and sodium, serum uric acid, serum creatinine (estimate glomerular filtration rate), microscopic evaluation of urine, microalbumin test and electrocardiogram.

Additional tests based on history, physical examination and routine laboratory findings: (ESH 2013). Glycated hemoglobin if fasting glycemia > 102 mg/dl or previous diagnosis of diabetes, quantitative proteinuria (if present in urine summary); urinary sodium and potassium and their ratio, ABPM (24-hour BP monitoring), echocardiogram, holter in case of arrhythmias, carotid ultrasound, peripheral and abdominal arterial ultrasound, ankle-brachial index, fundoscopy, pulse wave velocity and in resistant and complicated hypertension: testing for target organ damage and secondary hypertension when the history, laboratory tests and physical examination suggest it (ESH, 2013).

Physical examination. The aim is to establish a diagnosis of hypertension, assess secondary causes and estimate cardiovascular risk. All patients should undergo auscultation of the carotid arteries, renal arteries and cardiac auscultation with further investigation with carotid ultrasound, echocardiogram and renal artery doppler if murmurs are present. Height, weight and abdominal circumference should be measured with the patient standing and pulses should be palpated (ESH, 2013).

Signs on physical examination that suggest secondary hypertension. Aspects of *Cushing's Syndrome*, skin signs of neurofibromatosis (pheochromocytoma), palpation of abdominal masses (polycystic kidneys), auscultation of abdominal murmurs (renovascular hypertension), auscultation of the chest and thorax (coarctation of the aorta, arthritic disease, upper limb arterial disease), decreased or delayed femoral pulse (coarctation of the aorta, arthritic disease, lower limb arterial disease), difference in BP between the two arms (coarctation of the aorta, subclavian artery stenosis) (ESH/ESC, 2013).

Signs of damage to target organs (ESH/ESC, 2013).

Brain: sensory or motor defects; *retina:* abnormalities in the fundus; *heart:* third and fourth heart sounds, presence of cardiac murmurs, arrhythmias, location of the *ictus cordis;* pulmonary rales, *peripheral* edema; *peripheral arteries*: absence, reduction or asymmetry of pulses, cold extremities, ischemic skin lesions; *carotid arteries:* presence of murmurs.

Risk stratification (ESH/ESC, 2013).

FR/LOA/ DCV	Normal/High BP	HAS G1	HAS G2	HAS G3
Without FR		Low Risk	Mod. R.	High Risk
1-2 FR	Low Risk	Mod. R.	Mod/High R.	High Risk
>=3 FR	Bass/Mod. R.	Mod./High R.	High Risk	High Risk
LOA/IR/DM	Mod.R/High R.	High Risk	High Risk	High/M.High R.
DCV/IR/DM+ LOA	Very High R.	Very High R.	Very High R.	Very high R.

High R: high risk; CVD: Cardiovascular disease; DM: Diabetes mellitus; RF: Risk factor; G1:Grade 1; G2:Grade 2; G3:Grade 3; RI: Renal insufficiency; LOA: Target organ damage; Mod.R. (moderate risk); SAH: Hypertension; M.High R: Very high risk: BP: Blood pressure: R:Risk.

Follow-up according to risk stratification (ESH/ESC, 2013).

FR, LOA, DCV	BP nor - barely high	HAS G1	HAS G2	HAS G3
Without FR	No Intervention	SEM/months(?) Drugs if BP>140/90mmHg	SEM/weeks(?) Drug if BP>140/90mmHg	SEM Immediate Drugs
1-2 FR	SEM	SEM/week Drugs if BP>140/90mmHg	SEM/week Drugs if BP>140/90mmHg	SEM Immediate Drugs
>=3 FR	SEM	SEM/week Drugs if BP>140/90mmHg	SEM Drugs if BP>140/90mmHg	MEV Drugs Immediate
LOA/IR/ DM	SEM	SEM Drugs if BP>140/90mmHg	SEM Drugs if BP>140/90mmHg	SEM Drugs Immediate

CVD/symptom	SEM	SEM	SEM	SEM
s,IRC, or DM with LOA/FR		Drugs if BP>140/90mmHg	Drugs if BP>140/90mmHg	Immediate drugs

MEV: Lifestyle Change; CRF: Chronic Renal Insufficiency; RF - risk factor; LOA - target organ damage; DM - Diabetes mellitus; CVD - Cardiovascular disease.

Treatment (ESH/ESC, 2013).

Non-drug measures and the use of antihypertensive drugs are used with the aim of reducing BP and preventing damage to target organs, CV and renal outcomes. Non-drug measures are limited by loss of adherence in the medium and long term. Individuals with stage 2 and 3 hypertension and/or high risk (even in stage 1), or with BP ≥ 160/100mmHg should start drug treatment immediately. They can delay or prevent hypertension and reduce the number of doses of antihypertensive drugs, while also helping to control other risk factors and medical conditions. Measures include smoking cessation, salt restriction, moderate alcohol consumption, high vegetable, fruit and low-fat consumption, weight reduction and regular physical activity (DBHA, 2016).

Lifestyle changes should be suggested at the beginning of treatment, encouraged and reinforced over time. They have no known harmful effects, improve well-being, the response to drug treatment and are inexpensive (ROHRBACHER, 2014).

Salt restriction to 5-6 g/day is recommended. The effect is greater in blacks, the elderly, diabetics, patients with Metabolic Syndrome and kidney disease.

Hypertensive men should limit their alcohol consumption to 20-30g/day and women to 10-20g/day of ethanol (140g/week for men and 80g/week for women).

In terms of diet, it is recommended to eat vegetables, soluble fiber, reduce saturated fat and cholesterol, and eat fresh fruit. The Mediterranean diet has attracted widespread use because it recommends eating fish at least twice a week and 300-400g of fruit and vegetables (ESH, 2013).

The *Dietary Approaches to Stop Hypertension* (DASH) diet is recommended, rich in fruit and vegetables with low levels of total and saturated fat with exercise and weight loss. With regard to coffee, there is no consensus on whether it is harmful or beneficial (STESSEN, 2012).

Regular physical activity 5-7 times a week for a minimum of 30 minutes of moderate-intensity aerobic exercise (ESH, 2013).

With regard to drug treatment, there are several classes of drugs that are used according to the profile of the hypertensive patient and their comorbidities. Groups of drugs: beta-blockers, diuretics, calcium channel antagonists, angiotensin-converting enzyme inhibitors, angiotensin receptor blockers, renin inhibitors, alpha-blockers, central action agents and direct vasodilators (DBHA, 2016; 8th JOINT, 2014).

Acute and chronic complications of SAH (ESH, 2013):

Acute: Stroke, Acute Myocardial Infarction, Acute Aortic Dissection, Acute Pulmonary Edema.

Chronic: Chronic Kidney Disease, Congestive Heart Failure, Saccular Aortic Aneurysm, Left Ventricular Hypertrophy, Peripheral Arterial Disease, Carotid Atherosclerosis, Sexual Dysfunction, Arterial Stiffening.

Primary care - prevention and control of risk factors

Actions and strategies on risk factors (RF) are needed in order to prevent or delay the onset of SAH. They also involve general health promotion measures such as educational campaigns, recommendations, interventions and measures aimed at populations most at risk of developing the condition. Population action strategies focus on health promotion, focusing on education and knowledge about SAH and how to prevent it (BRANDÂO *et al*, 2012).

Strategies can be implemented through educational campaigns in print and electronic media, focusing on risk factors and lifestyle changes (LBM), the introduction of basic health notions in school curricula, the implementation of educational actions such as the National Day for Preventing and Combating SAH, actions in industries, religious organizations. These activities aim to raise awareness among the population of the need to adopt healthy habits in order to reduce, delay and even prevent the emergence of risk factors, resulting in a better quality of life and health (BRANDÂO *et al,* 2012).

These are complex actions, requiring the involvement of scientific societies, universities, organized civil society, entities formed by people with hypertension and the municipal, state and federal governments. The development of actions in communities and families is of the utmost importance and must be adapted to the cultural characteristics of each population and their diversity (DBHA; 2010).

The main risk factors involved in the genesis of hypertension are: age, family history of hypertension, excess weight, excessive alcohol consumption, excessive salt intake, sedentary lifestyle, black race, socioeconomic factors, genetics and those with pre-hypertension (KAVEY, 2003).

The adoption of primary prevention measures for hypertension in young people has been shown to be more effective, although it is desirable at any age. The identification of atherosclerosis in childhood, adolescence and young adulthood and the greater knowledge of the risk factors present in these age groups shows us the need to implement programs with the aim of early intervention in these RF (DBHA, 2016). There has been a large increase in childhood obesity and the percentage of children and adolescents diagnosed with SAH has doubled in the last twenty years (DBHA, 2016).

Educational measures should be established to reduce salt in food: avoid canned and preserved foods (peas, corn, hearts of palm, olives, pickles, asparagus), foods high in sodium (tomato extract, mayonnaise, tuna, sardines, sausages, cold cuts, salty cheeses, snacks, spices, sauces and ready-made broths, salted and industrially processed meats and industrialized soups) (BRANDÂO, 2012).

The Family Health Strategy (ESF) is the main form of primary care in Brazil's Unified Health System (SUS), where preventive measures must be implemented and monitored. It encompasses small and medium-sized municipalities (BRASIL, 2008).

After 20 years since the creation of the Family Health Program, there are currently (Jan/2014) 35,812 teams, distributed in 5,352 municipalities, covering 57% of the Brazilian population, which represents almost 111 million inhabitants. The PSF today is the Family Health Strategy (ESF), which sets it apart from selective programs and highlights its potential to build new forms of care, with better results in terms of health indicators themselves, as well as more ethics. It reveals that comprehensiveness can only be achieved to the extent that points of care of differing technological complexity are interconnected and communicate from a robust base - Primary Health Care (BRASIL, 2006; BRASIL, 2014).

Primary health care, as an integral part of the national health system, is the first element of a process of continuous health care that includes prevention, promotion, cure and rehabilitation, as established by the National Primary Health Care Policy of 2011 (SUMAR, 2014).

A meta-analysis evaluating adherence in cardiovascular disease included educational, behavioral and combined strategies. Behavioral strategies showed greater success than educational strategies. An important component is the patient's commitment to caring for their own health (SANTOS, 2013).

Despite the difficulties in adhering to treatment, advances in knowledge and developments in therapy have increased the population's life expectancy. With longevity, it is important that individuals maintain their autonomy and health, as ageing increases the risk of chronic diseases, especially cardiovascular diseases. Furthermore, with the increased survival of patients with chronic and/or serious illnesses, Quality of Life (QoL) has become more highly valued (CARVALHO, 2012; HOLT, 2013).

3. ADHERENCE TO TREATMENT - a strategy for controlling hypertension and preventing cardiovascular disease

Concepts and definitions

The word adesao comes from the Latin *adhaerere* which means to join, to join to, formed by a" and *haerere" to* join, to join to".

Adherence is also defined as the establishment of a joint activity in which the user is not a mere follower of medical advice, but understands and agrees with the recommended prescription; it is a dynamic, multidetermined process of co-responsibility between the user and the health team. It suggests an understanding of empowerment on the part of the person, making up a vision of the individual as an intra-active being, the result of their own inner dynamism, with the potential to express their peculiar way of being in the world (RIBEIRO, 2011).

Adherence to hypertension treatment is considered to be the coincidence between the user's behavior and the health professional's prescription, involving both pharmacological and non-pharmacological measures. Its aim is to control BP, reduce the incidence or delay the occurrence of cardiovascular complications and improve quality of life (SOUZA, 2008).

The terms used in the literature to define adherence and non-adherence are *compliance*, which can be translated as fulfillment and obedience, and more recently, *adherence,* translated as adhesion or ad*herence.* The term *compliance* suggests a passive role for the individual with SAH, originating from a doctor-centered paradigm and is more control-oriented (HALPERN, 2006). The term *adherence* identifies a free choice on the part of people who adhere or not to recommendations, with a certain collaborative interaction between the individual with SAH and the health professional (SANTA HELENA, 2007; SOUZA, 2008).

The WHO recommends using the term *adherence*, because the individual acts as a participant in the care process, in accordance with the therapeutic proposals of the health professionals.

Adherence to treatment is considered to be the patient's health-related behavior, more than just the act of using prescribed medication. The WHO defines it as the degree of a person's behavior in taking medication, following a diet and making lifestyle changes (LIMA, 2010).

In Brazil, non-adherence rates are: 49% in Rio de Janeiro, 43.4% in Porto Alegre, 86.3% in Sao Paulo, 25% in Sao Luiz and 36-42% in Fortaleza (BORGES, 2012).

The WHO cites that the magnitude and impact of low adherence in developing countries is even greater in view of the scarcity of health resources and inequalities of access (WHO, 2012).

Factors determining adherence

Adherence is therefore a complex behavioral process, strongly influenced by the environment, health professionals and medical care. Non-adherence is an impediment to achieving therapeutic goals and can be a source of frustration for health professionals. Mental disorders, depressive symptoms and loss of cognitive function are strongly associated with non-adherence (SANTA HELENA, 2010).

The WHO has established that several factors are involved in adherence to SAH therapy: those related to the patient: gender, age, ethnicity, marital status, education and socioeconomic level. Those related to the disease: chronicity, absence of symptoms and complications. They also involve health beliefs, lifestyle and cultural habits (perception of the seriousness of the problem, lack of knowledge, experience with the disease in the family context and self-esteem). There are also factors related to treatment and quality of life (costs, undesirable effects, complex therapeutic regimens). In relation to the institution, health policy, access to the health service, waiting time versus time to be seen. Finally, the factor related to interaction with the healthcare team (GUSMÂO, 2006).

Non-adherence is classically considered to be a complex and multidetermined phenomenon. Studies have shown that the rate of adherence to hypertension therapy decreases as time passes after the start of treatment. It is a condition of fundamental importance for the control of CNCDs such as SAH, as it is a pathology with a slow, long-lasting, continuous clinical evolution and the possibility of serious complications. Preventing and treating patients with hypertension involves a multidisciplinary approach with guidelines that are slow to implement and difficult to maintain. These actions must be permanent and patients must be motivated to adhere to them in order to achieve all the goals set (ALHALAIQA, 2012).

The belief that sufferers of this pathology are solely responsible for their treatment reflects a lack of knowledge about other factors involved that affect people's behavior and their ability to adhere to treatment. Those who have the support of friends or family are more likely to adhere to treatment, which is observed in chronic diseases all over the world (LACHAINE, 2008).

Proper understanding of the therapeutic regimen is a phenomenon associated with the patient's condition and is critical for medication adherence. Around 50% of patients who leave the clinic find it difficult to understand the proposed therapeutic regimen (GIROTTO 2013). A recent review on health literacy revealed that not understanding was associated with a higher chance of hospitalization, use of emergency services and, in the elderly, higher mortality (BERKMAN, 2011).

With regard to the use of medication, side effects are the biggest contributor to hindering adherence to SAH treatment. The medication regimen also has an influence, as the greater the number of tablets taken, the lower the rate of adherence to treatment. Individuals with comorbidities are also less likely to adhere to therapy, probably because of the care required and the number of drugs to be administered (MOLINA, 2006; HAMILTON, 2003; PLADEVALL, 2010).

There are various strategies for assessing adherence to hypertension treatment, but there is no gold standard (SANTA HELENA, 2007). The methods described in the literature are direct, such as the dosage of the active ingredient/metabolite of the drug, or indirect, such as counting pills and user reports.

Indicators of adherence to treatment

Progression of hypertension, prevalence of hypertension, attendance at appointments, use of medication, ability to maintain medication indefinitely, psycho-emotional conditions, commitment to health, absence of social support networks, forgetfulness and refusal of medication.

Controlled blood pressure / evolution of SAH.

The progression of hypertension is directly related to failures in adherence, leading to hospitalizations, deaths and sequelae (SOUZA, 2008). It is difficult to convince asymptomatic individuals that they are suffering from a chronic condition, leading to changes in lifestyle habits and the permanent use of medication (SOUZA, 2012).

Increased prevalence of SAH

Approximately 75% of people with hypertension keep their BP uncontrolled and of these, 1% develop one or multiple episodes of hypertensive crisis (HELENA, 2010).

Attendance at appointments and use of medication

They encourage adherence to treatment. The frequency of consultations and meetings between individuals and health professionals contributes to treatment adherence and BP reduction (TAMBLYN, 2010). In groups where meetings are frequent, there is greater maintenance of the reduction in blood pressure levels. There is a greater possibility of therapeutic adjustments, contributing to a more effective change in lifestyle, well-being and stress reduction (LACHAINE, 2008). The instruments that assess adherence focus more on drug treatment, revealing the correct use of medication, its monitoring and attendance at appointments, while greater emphasis is needed on lifestyle changes. There is often a lack of knowledge about hypertension and its treatment.

The complexity of the treatment regimen and its side effects contribute to a *poor* quality of life (SOUZA, 2007).

Psycho-emotional conditions.

Chronic environmental stress, the presence of depression, Parkinson's disease and deterioration in mental state contribute to failures in adherence to treatment (MENDOZA, 2006; LIBERTAD, 2007).

Ability to maintain treatment indefinitely.

It is related to knowledge about the pathology, the importance of controlling it and access to health services. It also involves the number of drugs administered, the complex dosage and their side effects. Because it is an asymptomatic disease with late complications, many people don't adhere to the recommendations, making it necessary to invest more in education and health (DBHA, 2016).

Commitment to health.

It is of the utmost importance to reflect on the influence that arises between the SAH user and the health professional. The concept of implied presence and presence in reserve is analyzed. The former refers to the act of constantly working with the individual and the latter refers to giving time and space to the other, not performing but remaining available without excessive intrusion. This implies an educational process, making them act as subjects, using their own knowledge and life experiences (DOURADO, 2011). There must be dialogue in care practices, with the aim of reducing distances, a conscious attitude of opening up the self in order to understand the other (ALHALAIQA, 2012).

Lack of social support networks and forgetfulness.

Low socio-economic status, low levels of schooling, unemployment, lack of effective social support networks, unstable living conditions, lack of access to basic healthcare facilities, cultural beliefs and little knowledge of the pathology and forgetting to take medication (PATEL, 2008).

Refusal of medication.

Side effects are the main contributor to non-adherence. The number of pills taken during the day also contributes (PATEL, 2008). Mainly because it is a chronic disease that requires long-term therapy and the fact that it is asymptomatic (DOURADO, 2011; MEDDINGS, 2012).

Family participation.

This is one of the most important determining factors in adherence to treatment, especially in the elderly. Support and the family context are essential in driving adherence to treatment, as well as in promoting the health of individuals with hypertension (MENDOZA, 2006).

In addition to medical consultations, other approaches are needed that can contribute to greater adherence. The work of the multidisciplinary team with the participation of the family creates spaces for individuals to verbalize symptoms, fears, insecurities, anxieties, frustrations and difficulties experienced in everyday life in relation to the disease and treatment. The group with family members stimulates reflection, increases the level of information and the exchange of experiences (ESTEVAN, 2013).

The social network that surrounds hypertensive patients has the role of encouraging positive personal attitudes in health monitoring, such as diet, physical exercise, sleep and adherence to drug treatment. The presence of the family transmits tranquillity, strength and courage, making them feel safe and supported in dealing with their pathology (COSTA, 2008).

Difficulty in adherence and lack of interest in treating hypertensive individuals occurs when the family is not involved in their daily care or when the relationship between family members is conflictual (COSTA, 2008).

The hypertensive's conscious attitude to adherence

Adherence involves several factors such as: attending appointments, regular use of medication, adopting a healthy lifestyle, and effective engagement in self-care activities (SANTOS, 2005; BOSWORTH, 2009). This involves raising user awareness through health education with the multidisciplinary team. The hypertensive patient must be involved and cooperate voluntarily, producing the desired therapeutic result (SANTOS, 2005; DIMATTEO, 2004; SANTOS, 2012).

It can be conceptualized as decision-making without sequelae or symptoms. It reflects the way in which health care is understood and assumed. The individual actively participates in all the recommendations given to them by health professionals. Active and voluntary participation in order to achieve their therapeutic goals (DOSSE, 2009; PERK, 2012; VAN, 2010).

Accepting and coping with the chronicity of this pathology involves understanding its meaning and conceptions of health and disease. Some patients declared to be non-adherent believed that hypertension was an intermittent pathology, requiring treatment only in the presence of symptoms (BLOCK, 2008).

The most effective therapy prescribed by the most careful doctor will control BP only if the patient is motivated to take their medication and self-establish health promotion measures with lifestyle changes (BURNIER, 2013).

Instruments and procedures for assessing adherence to treatment

Quantifying the lack of adherence to hypertension treatment is still a challenge for those dealing with this pathology, given the multifactorial nature of non-adherence. Direct indices for measuring adherence are intended to guide practice and point out probable flaws that should be addressed, facilitating the achievement of BP control targets (SANTOS, 2013). There is no gold standard for measuring adherence levels. Self-reporting, pill counting, electronic packaging, prescription renewals in closed pharmacy systems and serum medication levels have been used (FRANCO, 2013; LEANDRO, 2013).

Most existing tools focus only on drug treatment (OIGMAN, 2006).

Direct methods involve serial measurement of the drug level, are expensive and are not universally available. They have restricted access and are generally found in research laboratories, which contributes to the high use of indirect methods, which are simpler and lower cost, useful for clinical practice and can provide valuable information (LEANDRO, 2013).

Instruments that consider self-report are generally based on an epidemiological approach where the evaluation should be as accurate as possible. Most self-report questionnaires are more feasible, but have low sensitivity and high specificity (SANTA HELENA, 2008).

Health Belief Model (HCM)

Developed by social psychologists from the US health service in 1974 in an attempt to explain why people did not prevent themselves properly against diseases for which there were already tests or vaccines, such as tuberculosis and polio (SVARSTAD, 1999); ACOSTA, 2005; PIRES, 2008).

Electronic Tablet Counting (MEMS) (ZELLER, 2007).

The most reliable indirect method is electronic monitoring, which is widely accepted by patients and is effective in detecting "white coat adherence". However, like all methods, it has its limitations, especially in terms of the price of the device (KROUSEL-WOOD *et al.*, 2009). This method has been used in studies for 30 years and provides the researcher or clinician with data on the patient's drug-taking behavior (OSTERBERG and BLASCHKE, 2005).

Association between Medication Adherence and the 4-item Morisky Scale (MMAS-4).

As for the Morisky-Green scale of positive attitudes towards taking medication, developed in 1986, the fundamental theory of this measure is that inappropriate use of medication occurs in one, more than one, or all of the following ways: forgetfulness, carelessness, stopping the medication when feeling better or worse. It is easy to measure, validated, with only four comprehensible questions that provide verification of the person's attitude towards taking medication (MORISKY, 1986).

Association between Medication Adherence and the 8-item Morisky Scale (MMAS-8).

The MMAS-8, an update with greater sensitivity of the four items of the scale published in 1986 and considered the most commonly used self-reporting method for determining adherence, contains eight questions with closed dichotomous answers (yes/no) (OLIVEIRA, 2012; MORISKY, 2008).

Manual tablet counting (MCC)

Counting pills (e.g. counting the number of pills left in the patient's medication box) is a very simple method, but it is subject to problems such as the change of medication between boxes and the possibility of the patient discarding pills or capsules before the visit, in order to convince them that they are following the treatment (OSTERBERG; BLASCHKE, 2005).

Haynes-Sackett test

The Haynes-Sackett test is a methodology developed by Haynes and Sackett and consists of evaluating the average number of pills that the individual has forgotten to take over a period of time (HAYNES, 1980).

Medication Adherence Questionnaire - Qualiaids (QAM-Q)

It was developed to measure non-adherence to drug treatment in its many dimensions. It covers whether and how much the individual takes of their medication, how they take it over a seven-day period, whether they skip doses, whether they take it incorrectly, whether they take "holidays" and the result of adherence (in this case, whether their blood pressure was under control) (SANTA-HELENA; NEMES; ELUF-NETO, 2008).

Battle Test

The Batalla test is a test developed to check patients' knowledge of hypertension. It was later used as a predictor of adherence to treatment due to the strong correlation between adherence and knowledge (BATALLA-MARTiNEZ *et al.* 1984).

Questionnaire to assess adherence behavior to pharmacological and non-pharmacological treatment

This is a questionnaire used in its original version, which underwent a content validation process by *expert* nurses in Colombia using the indicators and the semantic scale of the NOC (*Nursing Outcomes Classification)* taxonomy as a reference (VELANDIA-ARIAS, 2009).

MBG (Martin-Bayarre-Grau) questionnaire

Developed at Cuba's National School of Public Health, it was based on the definition of therapeutic adherence developed by the authors: active and voluntary action by the user to adopt a behavior related to compliance with the treatment agreed upon in mutual agreement with their doctor. It is self-administered, short and easy to apply (ALFONSO, 2008).

Health Behavior Scale

It was used in a study in Chile. There is a modified scale to characterize adherence to treatment. Four subscales ask about diet, physical activity, taking medication and whether stressful situations can be controlled in each of the contexts in which daily life takes place (at home, in recreation and in social activities) and there is a fifth subscale that asks about smoking habits and extends to the workplace (MENDOZA, 2009).

Hill-Bone compliance to high blood pressure therapy scale. It assesses user behaviors across three important behavioral domains of high blood pressure treatment: 1) reducing sodium intake; 2) attending appointments; 3) taking medication. It was developed and validated by the John Hopkins University School of Nursing, Baltmoore, USA (KIM, 2000).

***Self-Reporting Questionnaire (SRQ-20)**:* (GARBER, 2004).

Created in 1986, it is used to screen for common mental disorders in primary care. The presence of mental disorders remains strongly associated with non-adherence to SAH treatment. The presence of depressive symptoms and loss of cognitive function are associated with non-adherence (MARI, 1986; GARBER, 2004).

Brief Medication Questionnaire (BMQ)

Created in 1999 to assess existing barriers to medication adherence. It asks which medications have been used in the last week (name, days, how many times a day, how many pills at a time, how many times the patient has forgotten to take a pill, whether the medication works well for the patient, regularly or not at all). If any medication is causing problems; he then evaluates a list of problems. At the end, he adds up the scores of the problems found.

Procedures for assessing adherence to treatment

Bromide method

The bromide method uses biological markers and calculates the concentration of the drug (or special biological markers added to the tablets) in the patient's blood or urine. This type of monitoring is accurate, but impractical in most clinical contexts, expensive and can in some cases be invasive (BUTLER; BRAAM, 2008).

Blood Pressure Measurement (BPM).

MPA is measured indirectly using a mercury or aneroid sphygmomanometer (VAN, 2010).

Arterial Blood Pressure Monitoring (ABPM)

In 1964, Hebert et al. demonstrated the benefits of ABPM and the possibility of assessing pressure during the patient's usual activities. The first publication demonstrating the possibilities of assessing 24-hour BP dates back to the 1960s. It is formally indicated in cases of suspected hypertension or the white coat effect (high BP in the clinic without or while taking medication). Its use is formally defined in the guidelines that standardize its use and in those conditions where there is doubt as to the real behavior of BP in casual measurements. BP during sleep can only be accessed by ABPM. It offers a unique possibility of analyzing the behavior between the 24-hour periods of vigilance and sleep. It consists of a recorder attached to the patient's waist and a cuff usually placed on the patient's left upper limb. The recording is made over 24 hours and the data is then transferred to a computer and analyzed using specific software (VII DBHA, 2016; RAY, 2012).

Home Blood Pressure Monitoring (HBPM).

ABPM is the recording of BP that can be done by taking three measurements in the morning, before breakfast and taking medication, and three in the evening, before dinner, for five days, or two measurements in each session for seven days, taken by the patient or another trained person, during surveillance, at home or at work, with validated equipment. Cheaper and easier to perform than ABPM, with limitations as it does not assess BP during sleep. It emerged after ABPM (DBHA, 2016).

The development of a specific instrument to measure adherence to treatment for hypertension must take into account its multidimensionality, focus on relevant aspects of this pathology associated with its therapeutic control and facilitate the detection and measurement of compliance with prescribed therapy. The creation of instruments is part of the development of health technologies. Technology is a process that involves different dimensions, resulting in a product that can be a durable good, a theory, a new way of doing something, or symbolic goods or products (ROCHA *et al.*, 2008; BEN, 2012).

4. HEALTH TECHNOLOGY - an instrument for social transformation

The etymology of the word technology: "tecno" derives from *techné,* which is know-how, and "*logia*" which comes from *logos* razao, meaning the reason for knowing how to do things. Technology can be classified into three types: Hard technology - machine-like equipment, instruments, norms, routines and organizational structures; - Hard light technology - structured knowledge, such as physiology, anatomy, psychology, clinical medicine, surgery, and Light technology - involves knowledge of the production of relationships between people. They are present in the user-worker space, and only materialize in acts such as welcoming, producing bonds, encounters of subjectivity and autonomy (MARQUES, 2010).

Technology can be defined, in a very simple and generic way, as applied knowledge. In the case of health, it is applied knowledge that enables the prevention, diagnosis and treatment of diseases and the rehabilitation of their consequences (VIANA, 2011; SILVA, 2003; SILVA, 2012).

Ordinance GM/MS n. 2.510, of December 19, 2005, which established the Commission for the Elaboration of the Technological Management Policy (CPG) within the scope of the SUS, defines health technologies as "medicines, materials and procedures, organizational, informational, educational and support systems, and assistance programs and protocols, through which health care is provided" (BRASIL, 2005). New technologies are constantly being incorporated into the SUS, which is a major incorporator of technologies that are of great importance for the health of the population. The National Health Technology Management Policy (PNGTS), approved in 2009, aims to maximize the health benefits obtained with the resources made available by the Ministry of Health (MS), ensuring that the population has access to effective and safe technologies, under conditions of equity (SILVA, 2012). It can be incorporated into goods (product technology) and/or be part of a process (process technology) (ROCHA, 2008; SILVA, 2012). As well as the National Policy for Science, Technology and Innovation in Health PNCTIS (2006), strengthening technological innovation and reducing external dependence (BRASIL, 2006).

It can't just be seen as something concrete, a tangible product, but as the result of work that involves a set of abstract or concrete actions aimed at health care. Technology involves the health work process, contributing to the construction of knowledge. It appears from the moment of the initial idea, the elaboration and implementation of knowledge and is the result of this same construction. It is both process and product (ROCHA, 2008).

Due to the current panorama of epidemiological and demographic transition with the predominance of chronic non-communicable diseases (CNCD) and the expansion of the elderly population, it is necessary to add new technologies and review the model of care practiced, prioritizing care acts and the autonomy of individuals (MALTA, 2010).

Incentives for research, development and innovation in health in Brazil have been included in the Organic Health Law since 1990. Specific scientific and technological policies in the health area were initiated in 1994. The 2004 National Policy for Science, Technology and Innovation in Health (PNCTIS) included Health Technology Assessment (HTA) among its strategies (VIANA, 2011).

HTA can be defined as a comprehensive way of researching the short- and long-term technical (almost always clinical), economic and social consequences of using health technologies, as well as their direct and indirect effects, both desirable and undesirable (VIANA, 2011).

The Postgraduate Program in Health Technology Assessment and Management established the Brazilian Network for Health Technology Assessment (REBRATS), with the aim of bringing together priority studies and research in the field of HTA, standardizing methodologies, monitoring the entry of new and emerging technologies, validating and attesting to the quality of the results to be disseminated to society. It was set up in August 2008 with the strategic vision of establishing links between research, policy and management to support the decision-making process, in a timely manner, in the phases of incorporation, monitoring and abandonment of technologies and technological innovation in health; represents the application of new knowledge, which can either appear in concrete form incorporated into a physical artefact (a piece of equipment, device or medicine, for example) or can represent "ideas", in the form of new procedures (or practices) or the (re)organization of health services (NOVAES, 2013). Its purpose is to promote and disseminate health technologies in Brazil.

The aim of REBRATS is to bring academic institutions and health services closer together in order to produce and systematize the information needed for decision-making on the incorporation of technologies into the SUS, the Ministry of Health and state and municipal health departments (NOVAES, 2000; NOVAES, 2013).

Chronic Non-Communicable Diseases (NCDs), such as SAH, are characterized by an uncertain etiology, multiple risk factors, long latency periods, prolonged course, non-infectious origin and are associated with functional disabilities. In recent decades, NCDs have become the leading cause of death in Brazil, accounting for almost 64% of deaths, far exceeding mortality rates from infectious and parasitic diseases (IPD). The epidemiological, demographic and nutritional transition has been taking place in Brazil, increasing the burden of NCDs, the elderly population and the accumulation of obese and overweight people, as well as other risk factors that predispose to increased morbidity and mortality from NCDs. There is an urgent need to articulate policies and programs aimed at tackling this reality, as well as to look more closely at the care that has been given to people with

CNCDs in health services, whether public or private. We need to reflect on care from the perspective of technology in order to improve the quality of life of people with hypertension (MALTA, 2010).

The work process in the Family Health Strategy (ESF) interacts with the user's knowledge and practices, inserting them as protagonists in the prevention, promotion and rehabilitation of health In order to establish health care relationships, applied knowledge is needed for this purpose, with the aim of guaranteeing it (MOREIRA, 2010).

The use of information and communication technologies is developing rapidly and is being used to increase adherence to treatment for chronic diseases such as hypertension. Of great importance is the use of technologies to promote communication between health professionals and patients. They focus on patient care and clinical information about the pathology. It aims to make patients more aware of the asymptomatic nature and chronic nature of hypertension and also helps to motivate adherence to pharmacological and non-pharmacological treatment. Effective medical education must be carried out continuously in order to result in behavioral changes. There is a great challenge in integrating all health professionals with patients to bring about these changes (SANTOS, 2013).

The National Program for Improving Access to and Quality of Primary Care (PMAQ), through the elements of Continuing Education, highlights the need to improve the organization of services and enrich the acquisition of knowledge and new technologies (PEDROSO, 2014).

Non-adherence to treatment is still a challenge to be overcome by health professionals together with users. The goal of these professionals is to engage them in self-care through health education strategies, with the aim of promoting and preventing health and consequently improving their level of health and quality of life (SANTOS, 2005).

Care is an axis on which we can think about building a cultural transformation of the social relationships that arise in the realization of health work, modifying the current practice in health services. The paradigm of care based on the material conditions of existence and the configuration of the health-disease process can refer to the essence of health work in the direction of the individual's integrality, which presupposes the commitment of health workers and users to jointly re-elaborate the care model (ALHALAIQA, 2012). An instrument for assessing adherence to hypertension treatment is a light technology that involves health knowledge and interaction between hypertensive individuals and health professionals.

5. METHODS FOR BUILDING AND VALIDATING TECHNOLOGY FOR ASSESSING HYPERTENSIVE USERS' ADHERENCE TO TREATMENT (TAT)

A methodological study of a quantitative nature. Polit, Beck and Hungler (2004) conceptualize a methodological study as one that investigates, organizes and analyzes data in order to construct, validate and evaluate research instruments and techniques, focusing on the development of specific data collection tools with a view to improving the reliability and validity of these instruments.

The study was carried out in the Primary Health Care Units (UAPS) distributed in the six Regional Health Coordinating Offices (CORES) of Fortaleza-CE. It should be noted that each SER contains between 11 and 20 Primary Health Care Units (UAPS). Therefore, 50.0% of the UAPS in each SER were randomly selected, which corresponded to 46, as shown in Chart 1.

Chart 1 - Number of existing and selected UAPS by SER.

COLORS	Existing UAPS	Selected UAPS
I	12	06
II	11	06
III	16	08
IV	12	06
V	20	10
VI	20	10
TOTAL	91	46

Source: Secretaria Municipal de Saùde (SMS) - Fortaleza-Ceara-Brazil.

In the state of Ceará, health care is organized into Macro-regions and Micro-regions of Health in order to comply with the doctrinal and organizational principles of the SUS (BRASIL, 2006; BRASIL, 2011a), which guides the process of decentralization of health actions and services and the processes of negotiation and agreement between managers. The Fortaleza macro-region is the largest in the state. It covers approximately 70.6% of the state's population, an estimated 6,032,600 inhabitants (SOUZA, 2013).

The municipality of Fortaleza-CE is divided into 6 (six) CORES - I, II, III, IV, V and VI. Each CORES is subdivided into several PAs (Private Areas), where superintendents, community leaders, secretaries and others work, with the function of guaranteeing a better life for the inhabitants and preserving the region's natural potential. Fortaleza-CE has 91 UAPS, 402 Family Health Teams

(EqSF), 2,458 Community Health Agents, 341 nursing assistants, 389 nurses and 369 doctors (Figure 1).

It should be noted that each UAPS has a Coordinator, the number of Family Health Teams (EqSF) varies according to the number of families registered and living in the area, and each EqSF is made up of a nurse, a doctor, a nursing assistant or technician, and at least six community health agents (ACS), depending on the size of the population assisted (Figure 1).

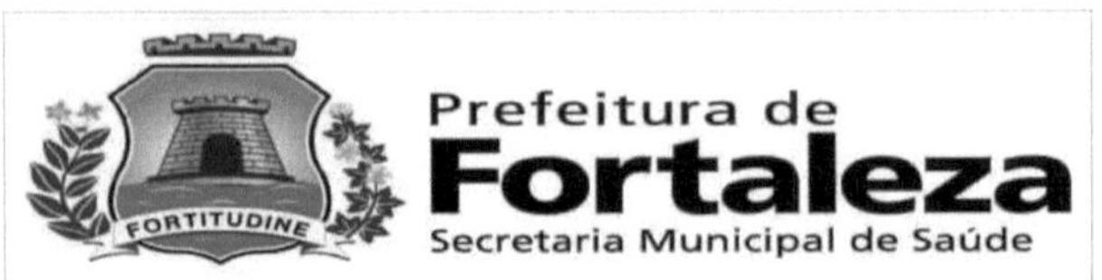

General Consolidation of Certificates, according to the month of JANUARY2014

BE	UAPS	No. Eq UAPS	No. of ESF doctors	N° ESF Enf	N° Aux Enf	NO. OF CHWS ESF
I	12	57	57	57	53	450
II	11	46	37	45	29	226
III	16	66	60	61	49	459
IV	12	41	35	41	41	225
V	20	89	86	87	87	565
VI	20	103	94	98	82	533
TOTAL	**91**	**402**	**369**	**389**	**341**	**2458**

Figure 1 - Distribution of UAPS and EqSF according to CORES

of the Municipal Health Department (SMS). Fortaleza-Ceara-Brazil.

Participating in the study were 71 (seventy-one) nurses and 39 (thirty-nine) doctors from the EqSFs located in the six CORES of Fortaleza-CE (Annex 1), who had been monitoring hypertensive users in the UAPS for 2 (two) years; and 10 (ten) judges who were doctors with extensive experience in monitoring people with *hypertension* and researchers on the subject of "*Adherence to hypertension treatment*".

It should be noted that the six CORES had 389 nurses and 369 doctors; and as for the judges, after electronic contact with 30 specialists, including nurses and doctors, only ten (10) of the doctors agreed to take part in the survey.

The following steps were taken to validate the TAT scores:

1°) The *Morisky-Green* instrument *(Appendix 2)* was *chosen* because it is more effective than the other instruments available to assess adherence to treatment (LEANDRO, 2013), in order to compare and adjust the TAT scores;

2) Application of the two instruments (TAT and *Morisky-Green (MG)* by the researcher in the selected groups of 80 (eighty) hypertensive users. When applying each instrument, the researcher assigned the same adherence parameters (TAT - excellent, good, fair, poor; *MG - low adherence, medium adherence and high adherence*), based on her experience in monitoring her hypertensive clientele.

3°) Comparison between the parameters achieved. There was no significant difference when comparing the results of the application of each instrument with those resulting from the researcher's experience. However, it was not possible to compare the results of the two instruments for two reasons: 1) MG evaluates "adherence" in only one modality of SAH treatment, while TAT evaluates it in both modalities; and 2) MG provides 3 (three) adherence profiles, while TAT provides 4 (four).

4°) Analysis and adjustment of the scores for validation purposes. Based on the comparative analysis of the instruments and the researcher's professional experience, the scores were kept a *priori.* Therefore, they could be altered or not by validating the EqSFs and the judges.

The TAT was validated by the EqSF (Nurses and Doctors) and by a Committee made up of 10 (ten) judges with extensive knowledge and experience in the field, in order to analyze the content, clarity and comprehension of the instrument (LOBIONDO - WOOD; HABER, 2001). The number of judges was in line with the recommendations of experts who suggest a minimum of five and a maximum of ten people (LYNN, 1986). As an inclusion criterion, it was recommended that the judges should have at least two (2) years' experience in monitoring hypertensive patients and be researchers on the subject of "*Adherence to hypertension treatment*". The "Committee of Judges" was therefore made up of 10 (ten) doctors.

To aid the process of validating the TAT, an *Instructional Guide for the Validation of the TAT* (GIAT) was constructed, based on the DBHA (2010) and an exhaustive review of the relevant literature.

This was followed by the validation study, for which the documents were sent to the EqSF and the judges: TAT; GIAT; TAT Evaluation Questionnaire (Appendix 1); Invitation Letter (Appendix 2); and Informed Consent Form (ICF).

Data was collected from July to September 2014 using the documents mentioned above. The list of judges was obtained from the website of the Brazilian Society of Hypertension and Cardiology, and only doctors and a registered nurse were found.

The data contained in the instruments answered by the FHTs and judges were organized and processed using the *Statistical Package for Social Science* (SPSS, version 20), represented in tables. The analysis of the results was based on analytical and descriptive statistics, using statistical tests in order to achieve the proposed objectives, especially the validity and reliability of the instrument. The analysis was based on the DBHA (2016), the European Guidelines and the relevant literature. It should be noted that the justifications in the participants' answers complemented the analysis of the quantitative data.

The research was carried out in accordance with Resolution 466/2012 of the National Research Ethics Commission (CONEP) (BRASIL, 2012), which regulates research with human beings. The FHTs and judges were guaranteed anonymity and the right to withdraw their consent at any time. The data was collected after the Free and Informed Consent Form (FICF) was signed and a favorable opinion was issued by the Research Ethics Committee of the University of Fortaleza - UNIFOR.

6. TECHNOLOGY FOR EVALUATING HYPERTENSIVE USERS' ADHERENCE TO TREATMENT (TAT)

The Technology for Assessing Hypertensive Users' Adherence to Treatment (TAT) was built based on the Brazilian Guidelines for Arterial Hypertension (2016) and consists of 4 (four) parts: Identification of the hypertensive user (IUH), Conducts for controlling hypertension (CCH), Indicators for Assessing Adherence to Treatment (IAT), and Profile of Adherence to Treatment (PAT), with their respective scores:

Part 1 - ***Identification of the hypertensive user (IUH). This*** consists of sociodemographic data such as age, gender, color, religion, profession/occupation, monthly income (in minimum wages), origin, place of birth, marital status, schooling, living conditions and who they live with.

Part II - ***Control of hypertension*** **(CCH*).*** The therapeutic behaviors inherent in the treatment modalities - basic and medication: 1. Healthy diet (0.0-20.0); 2. Regular physical exercise (aerobics) (0.0-20.0); 3. Regular use of medication (0.0-10.0); 4- Stress management (0.0-10.0); 5- Attendance at appointments with the EqSF (0.0-10.0); 6- Participation in health education activities (0.0-5.0); 7- Measurement of blood pressure (outside the clinic) (0.0-5.0); 8.Abstention from addictions - Smoking (0.0-10.0), Alcoholism (0.0-5.0), Others (illicit drugs) (0.0-5.0); 5. Therefore, the total sum of the scores will be from 0.0 to 100.0. The recording of these scores will be based on the user's report.

Part III - ***Indicators for assessing treatment adherence*** **(IAT)**. Controlled blood pressure (0.0-30.0), controlled weight maintenance (0.0-30.0), lipid profile within the established parameters (0.0-10.0), control of glycemic levels in diabetic users (0.0-20.0), and control of glycemic levels in non-diabetic users (0.0-10.0). Thus, the total sum of the scores will be from 0.0 to 100.0. These scores will be recorded on the basis of diagnostic methods and laboratory test results.

Part IV - ***Treatment Adherence Profile*** **(PAT)**. The PAT will be assigned based on the sum of parts I and II. Therefore, according to the sum achieved, the PAT will be: Excellent (160.0 - 200.0), Good (120.0 - 159.0), Fair (80.0 - 119.0), Poor (below 80.0).

Technology for Evaluating Hypertensive Users' Adherence to Treatment (TAT)

I Identification

1 Name 2.Age (years)

3. Gender ( ) Female ( ) Male 4. Color ( ) White ( ) Brown ( ) Black, ( ) Yellow 5. Religion ( ) Catholic ( ) Protestant ( ) Other

6. Individual monthly income (in minimum wages)7 Place of birth

8. monthly family income (in minimum wages)9. Origin

10. Profession/occupation ____

11. Marital status ( ) married ( ) single ( ) separated ( ) widowed ( ) other

12. Education ( ) Illiterate ( ) Literate ( ) Incomplete elementary school ( ) Complete elementary school ( ) Incomplete high school ( ) Complete high school ( ) Incomplete higher education ( ) Complete higher education

13. Housing conditions ( ) rented property ( ) own property ( ) other

14. Who do you live with ( ) children ( ) spouse ( ) other

II - SAH control measures

1. Healthy eating	***Intervals between scores***	**Scores** ***Found***
1.1 Proper use of salt	0,0 - 5,0	
1.2 Predominance of white meat (per week)	0,0 - 4,0	
1.3 Predominance of vegetables (per meal)	0,0 - 4,0	
1.4 Use of vegetable fat	0,0 - 3,0	
1.5 Proper use of coffee (up to 100ml/day)	0,0 - 2,0	
1.6 Use of dietary sweeteners	0,0 - 2,0	
2. ***Regular physical exercise (aerobics)***	0,0 - 20,0	
3. Regular use of the medication regimen	0,0 - 10,0	
4. *Stress management*	0,0 - 10,0	
5. Attendance at appointments with the EqSF	0,0 - 10,0	
6. Participation in health education activities	0,0 - 5,0	
7. Blood pressure measurement (out of office)	0,0 - 5,0	
*8. **Abstention of vices***		
8.1 Smoking ***If yes:***	0,0 - 10,0	

No. of cigarettes/day ________ Time of use (years) _______ ***If not:*** Never smoked ___________ Abstinence time (years)________ Time of use (years) ____________		
8.2 Use of alcohol ***If yes:*** Frequency of consumption ______________ Quantity consumed ____________________ Type of drink: Distilled ( ) Fermented ( ) Time of use (years) ***If no***: *Never used*___________ Abstinence time (years)__________ Type of drink: Distilled ( ) Fermented ( ) Time of use (years)	0,0 - 5,0	
8.3 Other (illicit drugs)	0,0 - 5,0	
Total scores	0,0 - 100,0	

III - Indicators for assessing adherence to treatment

Indicators*	***Scores Expected***	***Scores Found***
1. controlled blood pressure	30,0	
2. weight control	30,0	
3. Lipid profile within the established parameters	20,0	
4. control of glycemic levels	20,0	
Total scores	100,0	

*According to the current specific Brazilian Guidelines (Hypertension and Dyslipidemia)

IV - Treatment Adherence Profile (PAT)

Treatment Adherence Profile (TAP)	*Interval between Scores*	**Found score**	**PAT** Found
Excellent Good Fair Poor	160,0 - 200,0 120,0 - 159,0 80,0 - 119,0 Below 80.0		

7. instructional guide for the application of tat (giat)

I Presentation

The purpose of the Instructional Guide for the Application of the TAT (GIAT) is to contribute to the application of the **TAT.** The TAT was built based on the Brazilian Guidelines for Hypertension (2016), ESC/ESH,2013, DBD, 2013, and consists of Identification of the hypertensive user (sociodemographic data) and three (03) parts with their respective scores:

Part I - Control of hypertension (CCH)

The therapeutic approaches inherent in the treatment modalities - basic and medication: 1. healthy diet (0.0-20.0); 2. regular physical exercise (aerobics)

(0.0-20.0); 3. Regular use of medication (0.0-10.0); 4. Stress management (0.0-10.0); 5. Attendance at appointments with the EqSF (0.0-10.0); 6. Participation in health education activities (0.0-5.0); 7. Measurement of blood pressure (outside the clinic) (0.0-5.0); 8.Abstention from addictions - Smoking (0.0-10.0), Alcoholism (0.0-5.0), Others (illicit drugs) (0.0-5.0). Therefore, the total sum of the scores will be between 0.0 and 100.0. The recording of these scores will be based on the user's report.

1 Healthy eating

1.1 Proper use of salt. There is a relationship between the amount of salt ingested and BP levels. Although there are individual differences in sensitivity, the World Health Organization (WHO) has determined a maximum daily amount of table salt (sodium chloride) of 5 to 6g, which corresponds to 2g of sodium. Restricting this can reduce the number and doses of anti-hypertensive drugs. Therefore, avoid foods with a high sodium content, industrialized foods and sausages (ESH, 2013). In practice, this will be assessed by taste, since tasting salt in food implies that the amount is higher than recommended. It should be emphasized that alterations to the taste for salt occur with the time of high use of this compound, leading to the absence of its perception due to alterations in the taste buds, making them imperceptible to its high content, with desensitization occurring.

1.2 Predominance of white meats. White meats (fish and poultry without the leather) are low in animal fat and uric acid and are therefore healthier than red meats. You should eat them at least four times a week.

1.3 Vegetables predominate (fruits and vegetables). Vegetables contain both soluble and insoluble fiber. The recommendation is 20 to 30g/daily, with 5 to 10g insoluble. They help reduce weight and blood pressure (BP). 300 to 400g/day of vegetables is recommended (ESH, 2013). Fruit should be part of the 9am and 3pm snacks and dessert. The amount of vegetables in meals (e.g.

lunch) should be higher than the amount of carbohydrates.

1.4 Use vegetable fat. Monounsaturated fatty acids (oleic) such as olive oil, canola oil, olives, avocados and oilseeds (peanuts, chestnuts, walnuts, almonds) are recommended, and there is evidence that their consumption can reduce BP.

1.5 Proper use of coffee. The polyphenols contained in coffee have vasoprotective properties. In normal doses, caffeine does not raise BP (DBHA, 2010). Its effect on BP elevation is seen up to 30 (thirty) minutes after ingestion. However, there is no evidence in the literature of a long-term effect on BP (ESH/ECC, 2013). However, because they interfere with sleep quality, especially in the elderly, they can lead to the development of insulin resistance in the long term (CAUTER, 2011).

1.6 Use of dietary sweeteners. It is indicated for weight control, control of glycemic levels due to insulin hyperresistance in SAH, and glycemic control in diabetic users (FOSCAL2014).

2 Regular physical exercise

Regular aerobic exercise can be beneficial for preventing and treating blood pressure (BP), reducing cardiovascular risk and morbidity and mortality. It is advisable to do at least 30 minutes of moderate-intensity exercise 5 to 7 days a week. Recommended types of exercise are: cycling, walking, swimming, dancing and water aerobics (ESH/ESC, 2013). In addition to controlling BP, physical exercise combats obesity, dyslipidemia, insulin resistance and stress management.

4 Stress management

Emotional stress plays a role in triggering and maintaining hypertension, and can be a barrier to adherence to treatment. It can be managed through behavioral psychotherapy and the practice of meditation and *biofeedback* techniques, separately or together (DBHA, 2016). Stress is part of an individual's life, whether in the family environment or at work, and high stress loads stimulate the release of catecholamines with a consequent rise in BP.

5 Attendance at appointments with the EqSF

The consultation involves two fundamental moments for promoting the health of the hypertensive user: assessment of health conditions and adherence to treatment, and the second moment consists of the educational space, in which the professional will raise awareness and negotiate with the user about the conducts for controlling hypertension and the strategies for following them, in order to make them *excellent adherents*. According to current guidelines, 06 (six) are recommended

Nursing consultations (bimonthly) interspersed with 04 (four) medical consultations (quarterly).

6 Participation in health education activities

Health education activities should be carried out in groups with the aim of encouraging hypertensive users to adhere to treatment and involving family members in this goal, as well as investing in other actions to promote health and well-being.

<u>7 Blood pressure measurement (out of office).</u>

<u>8 Abstaining from addictions</u>

8.1 *Alcohol consumption.* There is a relationship between alcohol intake and BP levels depending on the amount ingested. There is controversy about the cardiovascular benefits of low doses. Acceptable - 30g of ethanol for men and 15g for women. Beer (6g/100ml), wine (12g/100ml), spirits (40g/100ml) (DBHA, 2016).

8.2 *Smoking.* Smoking is the greatest risk factor for atherosclerotic cardiovascular disease. It causes an acute rise in BP and heart rate (HR) for approximately 15 (fifteen) minutes after use. Smoking cessation should be encouraged. Its action is linked to the time of use and the number of cigarettes consumed.

8.3 *Illicit drugs.* The use of illicit drugs can also contribute to triggering hypertensive crises (DBHA, 2016). Acute BP elevation simulating pheochromocytoma can occur with cocaine use. Resistant SAH related to rapid and progressive renal failure can also occur. It has a powerful vasoconstrictive action on the renal arteries with fibrosis of the intima (AKKINA, 2012).

Part II - Indicators of Treatment Adherence (IAT)

Controlled blood pressure (BP) (0.0-30.0), controlled weight maintenance (0.030.0), lipid profile within the established parameters (0.0-10.0), control of glycemic levels in diabetic users (0.0-20.0), and control of glycemic levels in non-diabetic users (0.0-10.0). Thus, the total sum of the scores will be from 0.0 to 100.0. These scores will be recorded on the basis of diagnostic methods and laboratory test results.

<u>1 Controlled blood pressure (BP)</u>

PA is considered controlled according to the established parameters (DBHA, 2010; ESH/ECC, 2013).

Classification of hypertension (ESH, 2013). When systolic BP and diastolic BP are in different categories, the higher one should be used for classification. Normal-high BP or pre-hypertension are similar terms in the literature.

Classification of hypertension (ESH, 2013). Note: isolated systolic hypertension: SBP ≥140 and DBP < 90 mmHg

<u>2 Controlled weight maintenance</u>

There is an almost linear relationship between weight control and BP. Weight loss and a reduction in abdominal circumference (AC) are related to a reduction in BP and an improvement in metabolic status. Maintain a BMI of approximately 25 Kg/m^2 and an AC <102 cm for men and <88cm for women (DBHA, 2016).

3 Lipid profile within the established parameters (VI DBHA, 2016).

Targets according to cardiovascular risk		
Risk level	LDLC primary target (mg/dl)	Secondary LDLC target (mg/dl)
High	LDLC < 70	Non-HDL cholesterol<100
Intermediate	LDLC <100	Non-HDL cholestcrol<130
Bass	Individualized target	Individualized target

NOTE: People with low cardiovascular risk should receive individualized guidance.

Recommended levels (V BDD, 2013)		
Lipids	**Values (mg/dl)**	**Category**
	<200	Desirable
CT	200-239	Limited
	>=240	High
	<100	Great
	100-129	Desirable
LDL-C	130-159	Limited
	160-189	High
	>=190	Very high
HDL-C	>60	Desirable
	<40	Bass
	<150	Desirable
	150-200	Limited
TG	200-499	High
	>=500	Very high

Non-HDL cholesterol	<130	Great
	130-159	Desirable
	160-189	High
	>=190	Very high

4 Controlling glycemic levels in diabetic users

Non-pregnant users

Glycated hemoglobin	<7.0 g/dl
Fasting blood sugar	70-130 mg/dl
Postprandial blood glucose	<180 mg/dl

Source: American Diabetes Association (ADA, 2013).

NOTE: Postprandial blood glucose should be taken 1-2 hours after the start of the meal (ADA, 2013).

*Non-diabetic users (*ESH 2013)

Fasting blood glucose *less* than *or equal to* 99 mg/dl

Post-prandial blood glucose *below* 200 mg/dl.

Criteria for the diagnosis of diabetes mellitus (non-pregnant women) (ADA, 2013)

Glycated hemoglobin **greater than or equal to** 6.5%

Fasting blood glucose **greater than or equal to** 126mg/dl

Blood glucose **greater than or equal to** 200 mg/dl, 2 hours after 75g of glucose

Blood glucose **greater than or equal to** 200mg/dl in people with classic symptoms of hyperglycemia Source: American Diabetes Association (ADA, 2013).

Part III - Treatment Adherence Profile (TAP)

The PAT was adapted from the Self-Care Engagement Profile (PEAc) by Santos and Silva (2002). The PAT will be assigned based on the sum of parts I and II. Then, according to the sum achieved, the PAT is classified as: Excellent (160.0 - 200.0), Good (120.0 - 159.0), Fair (80.0 - 119.0), Poor (below 80.0).

Hypertension in the Elderly

1. In elderly hypertensive patients with SBP $\geq$ 160mmHg, it should be recommended to reduce

SBP to levels between 150 and 140 mmHg.

2. Physically well elderly people aged <80 years, start treatment for SBP values >140 mmHg with a target SBP <140 mmHg, if the treatment is well tolerated and the individual is in good clinical condition.

3. Elderly people over 80 with an initial SBP ≥ 160 mmHg are recommended to reduce their SBP to below 150 mmHg, provided they are in good physical and mental condition.

4. Frail elderly: it is recommended to leave decisions about antihypertensive treatment to the attending physician, based on monitoring the clinical effects of the treatment.

5. Continuation of well-tolerated antihypertensive treatment should be considered when a treated individual becomes octogenarian.

6. All antihypertensive agents are recommended and can be used in the elderly, although diuretics and calcium antagonists may be preferred in the treatment of isolated systemic hypertension.

8. Results of the validation process of the technology for ADHESION EVALUATION OF HYPERTENSIVE USERS TO TREATMENT - TAT

Characterization of the participants

According to Chart 1, the majority of FHTs (nurses and doctors) were women, aged between 20 and 39 years (52.7%), with academic training of between 10 and 19 years (48.2%), professional experience of between 8 and 13 years (42.7%), and postgraduate *latu sensu* specialization (51.8%).

As for the judges, they were predominantly female (70.0%), aged between 40 and 59 (80.0%), with between 20 and 29 years of academic training (60.0%), professional experience of 20 years or more (90.0%), and postgraduate studies - masters (40.0%) and doctorate (50.0%).

When considering a significance level of 5%, the hypothesis of equality between the characteristics of the EqSF and the judges was rejected, as follows: age range of 20 to 39 years in the EqSF; time since graduation for participants of 10 years or more; post-graduate course *latu sensu* (specialization) in the EqSF and *stritu sensu* (doctorate) in the judges; professional experience between 8 and 13 years only in the EqSF, over 20 years in the majority of judges (90.0%) and in 15.5% of the EqSF.

It was found that most of the professionals had only completed a *latu sensu postgraduate course,* although they had already completed eight years of training and professional experience, and that the career plan of the public institution to which they were attached included the gradual financial incentive inherent in postgraduate degrees.

There was a predominance of female professionals, which is probably due to the greater participation of women in the labor market since the 1970s, when more educated women got better jobs. This is due not only to economic needs and pressures, but also to the demographic, social and cultural changes that Brazil and Brazilian families have been going through since the middle of the 20th century. These include: a fall in the fertility rate, (II) a reduction in family size; an ageing population with a higher life expectancy at birth, although there is still a significant difference between women and men; and a sharp increase in family arrangements in which the reference person is female. The possibility of also working in the labor market has increased women's exposure to different ideals and contacts with other people beyond their family circle. Women's incomes have also come to influence their family decisions, often leading them to review their positions within their families (PINHEIRO, 2012).

Chart 1 - Distribution of FHTs (110) and judges (10) according to characterization. Fortaleza,

Ceará, Brazil, 2017. n = 120

Characterization	EqSF f	%	Ju f	izes %	p
GenderMale	20	18,2	03	30,0	0,40
Female	90	81,8	07	70,0	0,40
Age (years) 20-39	58	52,7	-	-	0,001
40-59	49	44,5	08	80,0	0,05
60 years or more	03	2,7	02	20,0	0,05
Training time (years) Less than 10	24	21,8	-	-	0,20
10 - 19	53	48,2	01	10,0	0,02
20-29	25	22,7	06	60,0	0,01
30 or more	08	7,3	03	30,0	0,04
Postgraduate studies					
Latu sensu Specialization	57	51,8	-	-	0,001
Residence	25	22,7	01	10,0	0,68
Strictu sensu Master's degree	20	18,3	04	40,0	0,11
Doctorate	-	-	05	50,0	0,0001
Length of experience (years) 02 - 07	22	20,0	-	-	0,20
08 - 13	47	42,7	-	-	0,006
14 - 19	24	21,8	01	10,0	0,68
20 or more	17 15,5		09	90,0	0,0001

$p < 0.05$ Significant

Validation of the Technology for Assessing Hypertensive Users' Adherence to Treatment (TAT)

The TAT consists of four parts: Identification of the hypertensive user (IUH), Behaviors to control hypertension (CCH), Indicators to Evaluate Adherence to Treatment (IAT), and Profile of Adherence to Treatment (PAT).

Identification of the hypertensive user (IUH)

The EqSF (100.0%) and the judges (100.0%) totally agreed with the hypertensive user identification data (UHI).

Socio-demographic data is of fundamental importance, in addition to identifying the user, in socio-economic and clinical assessment, diagnostic elucidation, early establishment of SAH control measures and those to prevent cardiovascular complications, assessment of adherence to these measures, as well as in the development of educational strategies to encourage adherence to treatment. It is worth noting that various socio-demographic data are related to the onset and complications of hypertension.

According to the Brazilian Society of Hypertension (SBH), the onset of hypertension and adherence to treatment can be directly influenced by several factors, including gender, age, ethnicity, education and socioeconomic status (DBHA, 2016). There is a direct relationship between blood pressure (BP) and age, with a prevalence of over 60% in individuals over the age of 60. Prevalence is higher in men up to the age of fifty, with an inverse relationship observed from this age group onwards. With regard to color, it predominates in non-white individuals, but we don't know for sure the effect of miscegenation in our society, which is why we don't refer to color. There is also a higher prevalence of individuals with low socioeconomic status and less schooling (MARTINEZ, 2006).

Several comparative studies between men and women show that men are more vulnerable to illness, especially serious and chronic illnesses. And they don't seek out primary care services in the same way as women. Chronic treatments are generally less adherent, as the therapeutic regimens require a great deal of commitment from the patient and lifestyle changes in order to complete the treatment. This is true for health promotion and prevention actions, which require behavioral changes (BRASIL, 2009).

Marital status also has a major influence on adherence to treatment for hypertension, since family support is fundamental, especially for the elderly, for this to happen. With regard to family support, individuals who share experiences with their spouses and receive support from them may have better participation in following treatment, but those who do not live with their spouse and live with children or other people have lower adherence to the therapeutic regimen (MENDES, 2014).

The participation of the family is fundamental in stimulating self-care. Their spouses are a crucial facilitator of treatment and its continuity.

Control of hypertension (CCH)

According to Table 2, the EqSF totally agreed with the CCH, ranging from 83.6% to 89.1%, and the judges from 60.0% to 100.0%.

However, the CCHs were partially accepted by the EqSF in a range of 10.0% to 14.5%, and by the judges in a range of 10.0% to 40.0%, except for (a): regular physical exercise, use of a medication regimen, stress management, abstention from smoking and alcohol use, and other addictions (illicit drugs). For the EqSF, it would be necessary to record the time and frequency of physical exercise in the TAT; and for the judges, to record the type of drug (illicit) and the time of use (if yes). It should be noted that this information can be found in the GIAT.

[...] *it is important to add the time and frequency of physical exercise to the TAT* [...] (E22)

[...] *in the item "other drugs" put the type of drug and time of use, if yes* [...] (J9)

The practice of physical exercise follows the recommendations of the DBHA (2010), which is based on the protocols of the *American Hearth Association* (AHA) and the European Guidelines.

Among illicit drugs, cocaine is the one that causes the most cardiovascular alterations. It induces intravascular thrombosis, hypertensive crises, a rise in BP and heart rate through alpha-adrenergic stimulation and is dose dependent, with endothelial dysfunction occurring over time (SCHUARTZ, 2010). It also causes left ventricular hypertrophy, left ventricular systolic and diastolic dysfunction and arrhythmias. It is usually consumed concomitantly with other drugs such as alcohol and cigarettes, which can exacerbate its harmful effects (MACEIRA, 2014). There is an association between the use of illicit drugs and risk factors for cardiometabolic diseases, especially cardiovascular disease (CVD) and type 2 *diabetes mellitus* (VIDOT, 2013).

Holiday *Heart* Syndrome is described when alcohol abuse occurs and appears to increase BP, leading to hypertension, which in itself is a risk factor for other CVDs and sudden death. It is also associated with procoagulant changes after acute intake, hypocoagulation with chronic abuse, and thrombocytosis after withdrawal. It can also reduce cerebral blood flow and cerebral metabolism due to chronic abuse or lead to vasoconstriction of the cerebral arteries with acute ingestion. It also causes arrhythmias and can lead to cardiomyopathy (TONELO, 2013).

The FHT in a range of 0.9% to 2.7% disagreed with the CHCs, with the exception of regular physical exercise, stress management, attending appointments with the FHT, and taking part in educational activities. As for the judges, only one (10.0%) disagreed with each of the CCH - regular physical exercise, regular use of the medication regimen and stress management.

The EqSFs recommended recording the time and frequency of physical exercise on the TAT; and the judges suggested defining "stress management", recording the type of drug (illicit) and the time of use (if yes), and also the time and frequency of physical exercise. This information is contained in the GIAT and is intended for consultation by the EqSF.

[...] *it is important to add the time and frequency of physical exercise to the TAT* [...] (J2)

[...] *it would be enlightening to define "stress management", since stress is a risk factor for SAH and something we experience on a daily basis* [...] (J1)

Epidemiological studies have shown that regular aerobic exercise can be beneficial for the prevention and treatment of hypertension, thus helping to reduce mortality. At least 30 minutes of aerobic exercise should be practiced five to seven times a week, reducing BP and improving other metabolic parameters (ESC/ESH, 2013).

Managing stress in everyday life means knowing how to deal with it, using relaxation techniques such as music therapy, yoga, meditation and leisure, and above all avoiding contact with stressors if possible. Stress can be reduced through stress management techniques, which are resources available for dealing with stress. Stress results from a lack of or ineffective adaptation, i.e. a person's ability to cope with it is reduced. There are various techniques for managing stress, such as cognitive techniques, problem-solving training, relaxation techniques (the most widely used) and self-instruction training (replacing stress-provoking thoughts with positive ones) (SOUSA, 2014).

Regularly attending appointments with the health team is a strategy for getting hypertensive patients to adhere to the program, provided that they and their families are encouraged to do so. The consultation involves two key moments: an assessment of health conditions through the presentation of the person's complaints and a physical examination; and an educational moment which aims to prepare both the person and their family for self-care (SANTOS and SILVA, 2002), leading to adherence to measures to control hypertension and prevent associated cardiovascular complications and other problems, thus contributing to the promotion of their health and well-being.

In general, the family is the first health unit that its members use and its characteristic is the ability to detect signs of abnormality in its individual. The fact that family members are always in close proximity, or that they have a routine and live together, gives them the opportunity to participate more actively as agents of care. Therefore, it can be seen that the family must be closely involved in the client's care and adherence to treatment, given their decision-making nature and their intimacy with the client, which takes place through daily life, i.e. activities of daily living, where the family member is present and participates in the whole process, from simply preparing the client's meal to going to appointments with the client.

Multiprofessional care should start from the user's first contact with the health service and be perpetuated. Motivational and educational techniques should be used, even when the team is restricted, as is seen in most existing UAPS where there are only doctors and nurses (NASCIMENTO, 2010).

Participation in educational activities" enables hypertensive users to adhere to their treatment and can make them multipliers of these actions among their families.

The "measurement of BP" outside the clinic is of great importance, as it provides a large number of measurements outside the institutional environment, and therefore a more accurate assessment of BP. It is verified through Ambulatory BP Monitoring (ABPM), Self-Measured BP (SMA) or Home BP Monitoring (HBPM). ABPM may not be feasible if the person has cognitive *impairment*, physical limitations, anxiety or obsessive behavior (DBHA, 2010).

Smoking among hypertensive people causes an acute increase in BP and heart rate (HR), which persists for more than 15 (fifteen) minutes with an increase in plasma catecholamines and impairment of the baroreflex. It is a powerful risk factor for CVD (ESC/ESH, 2013). As previously described, among illicit drugs, cocaine use has a thrombogenic action and also causes an acute rise in BP.

There is a linear relationship between alcohol consumption and elevated BP and the prevalence of hypertension. Total consumption should not exceed 140g per week for men and 80g per week for women (DBHA, 2010).

Chart 2 - Distribution of FHTs (n = 110) and judges (n = 10), according to responses related to SAH Control Conducts (CCH). Fortaleza- Cearà-Brazil, 2017. n = 120

Answers	Totally agree					Partially agree					I disagree				
	EqSF		Judges			EqSF		Judges			EqSF		Judges		
rol of hypertension (CCH)	f	%	f	%	p	f	%	f	%	p	f	%	f	%	p
Healthy eating															
Proper use of salt	93	84,5	06	60,0	0,08	16	14,5	04	40,0	0,06	01	0,9	-	--	1,00
Predominantly white meat[1]	95	86,4	08	80,0	0,63	12	10,9	02	20,0	0,33	03	2,7	-	--	1,00
Predominantly vegetables[2]	96	87,3	08	80,0	0,62	13	11,8	02	20,0	0,61	01	0,9	--	--	1,00
Use of vegetable fat	96	87,3	08	80,0	0,62	13	11,8	02	20,0	0,61	01	0,9	--	--	1,00
Proper use of coffee[3]	95	86,4	09	90,0	1,00	13	11,8	01	10,0	1,00	02	1,8	---	----	1,00
Use of diet sweeteners	98	89,1	09	90,0	1,00	11	10,0	01	10,0	1,00	01	0,9	---	----	1,00
Regular physical exercise	96	87,3	09	90,0	1,00	14	12,7	01	10,0	0,60	--	--	01	10,0	0,08
Regular use of medication	92	83,6	09	90,0	1,00	16	14,5	-	-	0,35	02	1,8	01	10,0	0,23
Stress management	94	85,5	09	90,0	1,00	16	14,5	-	-	0,35	--	--	01	10,0	0,08
Attendance at appointments	98	89,1	09	90,0	1,00	12	10,9	01	10,0	1,00	--	--	--	--	1,00
Participation in educational activities	96	87,3	09	90,0	1,00	14	12,7	01	10,0	1,00	--	--	--	--	1,00
Blood pressure measurement[4]	96	87,3	09	90,0	1,00	13	11,8	01	10,0	1,00	01	0,9	--	--	1,00
Abstention from vices:															
Smoking	95	86,4	10	100,0	0,36	14	12,7	-	-	0,60	01	0,9	--	---	1,00
Alcohol use	96	87,3	10	100,0	0,60	13	11,8	-	-	0,60	01	0,9	--	--	1,00
Others	97	88,2	10	100,0	0,60	12	10,9	-	-	0,60	01	0,9	--	--	1,00

$p < 0.05$ Significant [1] Per week [2] Per meal [3] Up to 100ml/day [4] Out of office

At a significance level of 5%, the hypothesis of equality between the opinions of the EqSF and the judges in relation to SAH control measures was not rejected. This means that the participants maintained the same position on these measures, including the scores.

Indicators for assessing adherence to treatment (IAT)

In Table 3, the majority of EqSF (89.1% to 92.7%) and judges (80.0% to 90.0%) totally agreed with the IAT. However, in a percentage range of 6.4% to 9.1% for the EqSFs and 10.0% to 20.0% for the judges, there was partial agreement with the IATs.

IATs are of fundamental importance for assessing hypertensive users' adherence to treatment. According to the DBHA (2016), controlled BP is directly related to weight control, glycemia and normal blood lipid parameters. With these indicators under control, there is less chance of atherosclerosis developing, and consequently of damage to target organs. The role that target organ damage plays in determining cardiovascular risk is crucial. These are asymptomatic lesions that gradually develop and compromise the heart, blood vessels, kidneys and brain.

In SAH risk stratification, diabetics are considered to be at high or very high risk of cardiovascular events. Type 2 *diabetes mellitus* has a 3 times greater chance of developing coronary heart disease and the individual with chronic hyperglycemia, 2 times more compared to the non-diabetic. Insulin resistance has also been cited as a predisposing factor to atherosclerosis. There is a concomitant reduction in HDL-c levels, an increase in LDL-c and visceral obesity. Hyperinsulinemia and insulin resistance at the vascular level also contribute to vascular injury and the atherosclerosis process. Controlling these factors - hyperglycemia, HDL-c and LDL-c levels and BP - is important to protect against the onset of atherosclerosis in diabetics (PANENI, 2014).

The main determinants for the onset of *diabetes mellitus, in* addition to genetic factors, are obesity and a sedentary lifestyle, which can be prevented through lifestyle changes and a reduction in body weight (DBHA, 2016).

High BP is associated with the risk of acute complications such as acute coronary syndrome, acute pulmonary edema, hypertensive encephalopathy, stroke, acute aortic dissection and chronic complications such as peripheral vascular disease, kidney failure, heart failure, chronic aortic dissection and saccular aortic aneurysm (DBHA, 2016).

On the other hand, obesity, especially abdominal or central obesity, plays a major role in the development of metabolic syndrome, with insulin resistance being the main factor. Metabolic syndrome is made up of abdominal obesity, changes in lipid profile, high blood pressure and hyperinsulinemia, which can evolve into *diabetes mellitus, the* development of CVD and insulin resistance. Adherence to lifestyle changes such as weight loss and weight control is essential for treating this condition (SANTOS, 2013).

SAH is closely related to excess weight. Maintaining a body mass index (BMI) of around 25 kg/m^2

and an abdominal circumference of 102 cm for men and 88 cm for women is included in the current guidelines (DBHA, 2016; ESC/ESH, 2013).

Higher scores were established for controlled BP and controlled weight maintenance, as they require greater engagement and adherence to the CHC, and greater commitment on the part of the hypertensive individual.

The *Dietary Approaches to Stop Hypertension* (DASH), rich in fruit, vegetables, fiber, minerals and low-fat dairy products, has an important impact on reducing BP. A high degree of adherence to this type of diet reduced the development of hypertension by 14%. The benefits on BP have been associated with a high intake of potassium, magnesium and calcium. It also enhances the effect of nutritional guidelines for weight loss, reducing biomarkers of cardiovascular risk (SACKS, 2001).

SAH is common in diabetics. Controlling blood glucose levels protects against the development of cardiovascular and ocular complications and diabetic nephropathy. These individuals should be counseled, as most of them are unaware of these complications.

At a significance level of 5%, the hypothesis of equality between the opinions of the EqSFs and the judges with regard to the IATs was not rejected. Therefore, the opinions of the participants were congruent in relation to the IAT.

Chart 3 - Distribution of EqSFs (n = 110) and judges (n = 10) according to their responses to the TAT's Indicators for Assessing Adherence to Treatment (IAT).

Fortaleza- Cearâ-Brazil, 2017. n = 120

Answer	Totally agree					Partially agree				
	EqSF		Judges			EqSF		Judges		
Indicators for Assessing Adherence to Treatment (IAT)	f	%	f	%	p	f	%	f	%	p
Controlled blood pressure	101	91,8	09	90,0	0,60	09	8,2	01	10,0	1,00
Controlled weight management	99	90,0	08	80,0	0,30	11	10,0	02	20,0	0,30
Lipid profile within established parameters	102	92,7	09	90,0	0,55	08	7,3	01	10,0	0,55
Controlling blood sugar levels (diabetic users)	100	90,9	08	80,0	0,26	10	9,1	02	20,0	0,23
Control of glycemic levels (non-diabetic users)	98	89,1	09	90,0	1,00	12	10,9	01	10,0	1,00

$p < 0.05$ Significant

Treatment Adherence Profile (TAP)

According to Table 4, the classification and scores assigned to the PAT were totally and unanimously agreed upon by the judges (100.0%). As for the EqSF, 94.5% totally agreed with the PAT. However, 6 (5.4%) partially agreed with the classification.

Chart 4 - Distribution of FHTs (n = 110) and judges (n = 10), according to answers related to the classification of the PAT. Fortaleza-Cearà-Brazil, 2017. n = 120

Answer	I totally agree					Partially agree				
	EqSF		Judges		p	EqSF		Judges		p
Treatment Adherence Profile (TAP)	f	%	f	%		f	%	f	%	
Excellent	104	94,5	10	100,0	1,00	06	5,4	-	-	1,00
Good	104	94,5	10	100,0	1,00	06	5,4	-	-	1,00
regular	104	94,5	10	100,0	1,00	06	5,4	-	-	1,00
Evil	104	94,5	10	100,0	1,00	06	5,4	-	-	1,00

$p < 0.05$ Significant

According to the 5% significance level, the hypothesis of equality between the opinions of the EqSF and the judges regarding the PAT (classification and scores) was not rejected. Therefore, it appears that the participants' opinions were in agreement regarding the PAT.

A hypertensive user with an Excellent PAT implies that he or she is strictly following the CCH, and that the targets for achieving optimal BP control are met by evaluating the indicators of adherence to treatment in the range of 80.0-100.0% of the total TAT scores, with consequent promotion of his or her health and a better prognosis and lower risk of developing cardiovascular complications.

The hypertensive user with Good PAT was able to adhere largely to the CCH and the targets of the treatment adherence indicators in the range of 60.0-79.5% of the TAT scores, through health promotion measures and with a good prognosis.

The hypertensive user with regular PAT was able to adhere to CCH of around 40.0-59.5% of the TAT scores, by evaluating adherence to health promotion measures and the predicted targets of the indicators for health promotion measures with regular prognosis.

Hypertensive users with poor PAT followed the CCH, reaching up to 40.0% of the TAT scores, with a higher risk of developing cardiovascular complications and a worse prognosis.

SAH is considered the biggest public health problem in developed and developing countries, either because of its high prevalence in the adult population or because it is considered the main risk factor for CVD. Adherence to treatment for hypertension is one of the biggest challenges for health professionals, as 40% of hypertensive patients do not adhere satisfactorily to treatment. The main causes of non-adherence to hypertension treatment are the complexity of the treatment regimen, length of treatment, failure of previous treatment, frequent changes in treatment, influence on quality of life, beliefs, lack of knowledge on the part of the patient and the relationship with the health team. Non-adherence to antihypertensive treatment can lead to serious cardiovascular complications, such as coronary heart disease, heart failure and stroke. CVD is responsible for 27.0% of deaths in Brazil and is one of the biggest causes of morbidity and mortality in the Western world. This high incidence can be explained by the high prevalence of SAH in the Brazilian population. In Brazil, stroke deserves to be highlighted for being the main cause of hospitalizations, mortality and sequelae, surpassing even other heart diseases and cancer (MENDONÇA, 2012).

Health professionals should monitor hypertensive patients regularly, providing them with lifelong guidance on the disease and treatment through health education, with the aim of preventing complications. Such follow-up is necessary, since adherence to treatment for hypertension is a complex process and must be constant because it requires the involvement and active participation of patients in practicing self-care, with a view to preventing diseases and promoting health (MENDONÇA, 2012).

In terms of gender, men are more vulnerable to diseases, especially serious and chronic ones. Despite their greater vulnerability and high morbidity and mortality rates, men do not seek out primary care services in the same way as women. Chronic or long-term treatments generally have lower adherence rates, since the therapeutic regimens require a great deal of commitment from the patient who, in some circumstances, needs to change their lifestyle habits in order to comply with the treatment. This is also true for health promotion and prevention actions, which most often require changes in behavior (MENDES, 2014).

Chronic non-communicable diseases such as SAH generate a high social and economic burden on the Brazilian public health system, since of the 7 billion reais spent on hospitalizations by the SUS in 2006, approximately 3 billion were spent on paying for hospitalizations for these causes. In addition, the majority of sickness benefits and early disability pensions are due to this group of illnesses, especially for young and middle-aged people between the ages of 20 and 60 (PIMENTA, 2012).

Disease prevention and health promotion are tools used to deal with these diseases. The first refers to interventions on risk factors in order to prevent the onset of specific diseases, reducing their incidence and prevalence in populations. The second refers to broader measures, lifestyle changes that aim to provide general health and well-being (PIMENTA, 2012).

General evaluation of the TAT

According to Table 5, the overall evaluation of the TAT was satisfactory for most of the EqSFs and judges, i.e. the EqSFs positioned themselves in a percentage range from 73.6% to 100.0% and the judges from 60.0% to 100.0%.

Based on the significance level of 5%, the hypothesis of equality between the opinions of the EqSFs and the judges with regard to the constituent items of the General Assessment of the TAT was not rejected. Therefore, it can be seen that there was a consensus in the positioning of the participants in the General Assessment of the TAT.

Chart 5 - Distribution of EqSF (n = 110) and judges (n = 10), according to the General Evaluation of the TAT. Fortaleza, Ceará, Brazil, 2017. n = 120

General evaluation of the TAT	EqSF		Judges		
	f	%	f	%	p
Feasibility and Applicability	95	86,4	09	90,0	1,00
Inherent aspects of treatment modalities	110	100,0	10	100,0	1,00
Aspects inherent in adherence to SAH treatment	99	90,0	08	80,0	0,30
Modifications or additions to the TAT					
- *Control of hypertension*	34	30,9	04	40,0	0,72
- *Aspects of adherence to treatment*	20	18,2	04	40,0	0,11
- *Agreed scores*	29	36,4	04	40,0	0,46
- *Adherence indicators (IAT)*	14	22,7	02	20,0	0,62
- *Treatment Adherence Profile (PAT)*	03	11,8	-	-	1,00
- *Instructional Guide (GIAT)*	13	21,8	03	30,0	0,13

$p < 0.05$ (Significant)

Feasibility/Applicability of TAT

For 95 (86.4%) FHTs, the TAT was feasible/applicable due to its objectivity and conciseness, the fact that it could be incorporated into nursing consultations, the fact that it helped promote the health of hypertensive patients, the fact that it provided subsidies for drawing up a care plan, and the fact that it encouraged FHTs to reflect on integrated care for hypertensive patients.

[...] it's *very feasible because primary care is the ideal place to assess adherence to treatment and it's easy to apply because it's objective and concise. I think its applicability during consultations in primary care is quite feasible* [...] *and primary care is the ideal place to assess adherence to treatment* ... (E16, E20)

The ideal place to establish measures for the prevention and early detection of hypertension is Primary Health Care (PHC), through the Family Health Strategy (FHS). It can be addressed through lifestyle changes and/or drug treatment with antihypertensive drugs, depending on risk stratification. Promoting strategies that enable adherence should be a goal of the EqSF (FAJARDO, 2010).

[...] *it's a good proposal for assessing adherence to the treatment of users with hypertension. It's an instrument that's easy to apply without taking up too much time in the consultation, with simple and direct questions that can be incorporated into the consultation* [...] (M9, E17)

The purpose of the TAT is to evaluate the hypertensive user's adherence to treatment, identifying the aspects that may require intervention by the health team so that the individual achieves the best possible PAT, thus contributing to a reduction in the rate of cardiovascular morbidity and mortality related to hypertension.

[...] *the TAT proposal is very good, it covers all the aspects for promoting the health of hypertensive users* [...] *the problem I see is the short time it takes to cover the whole instrument (TAT)* (M33)

Health promotion is carried out through programs and actions that focus on health rather than disease. It involves investing in quality of life, in which the individual is seen as a whole, with their cultural, historical and social aspects. Promoting health means taking action to create favorable conditions for the full development of human potential. This involves the individual, the family, the community, managers and health professionals. The EqSF is the model, because its object is health promotion and not the disease (source).

In SAH, there are non-modifiable risk factors such as age, heredity, gender and ethnicity/race, and modifiable factors such as clinical, behavioral and nutritional. Health promotion strategies are needed to address these modifiable factors, reducing the risk of complications, bringing individual and collective benefits for preventing SAH and reducing complications and chronicity (SALOMÂO, 2013).

[...] an *interesting proposal, as it provides us with subsidies for identifying vulnerability and drawing up a care plan* [...] *however, professionals have to reflect on the importance of its applicability for the benefit of hypertensive patients* [...] (E1, E68)

The work of the EqSF enables knowledge of the social reality and the socio-economic, food, health and family conditions of the communities, facilitating the primary care action strategy. Its aim is to detect what is preventing greater adherence to hypertension treatment, forming partnerships between hypertensive people and their families, establishing group and/or individual educational actions through a self-care plan (MIRANZI, 2008).

[...] *it's viable for assessing the level of adherence of hypertensive patients to treatment, because we always assess mainly the level of blood pressure and adherence to medication. With this tool, care will always be complete* [...] (E21)

The WHO defines adherence to the treatment of chronic illnesses as a multidimensional phenomenon, involving five factors, called dimensions: the health system, the disease, the treatment, the individual and the caregiver.

Some professionals who admitted the feasibility/applicability of the TAT, linked it to certain conditions: implementation of the TAT through electronic means, planning in the care of hypertensive people for the inclusion of the TAT, and availability of the necessary FHT to meet demand.

[...] it's *only feasible to apply it in practice if it (T, AT) is implemented in the computer program used by us in the town hall. Otherwise, if it's just on paper, it won't go any further [...*] (E31)

New technologies are being used in healthcare, including the use of software and electronic medical records, in accordance with CFM Resolution 1638/200. The purpose of health information is to integrate clinical and administrative data in order to optimize and qualify care, reduce costs and obtain relevant information that makes up a health profile in a given region. The Electronic Patient Record (EPP) is an important tool that healthcare staff use in their daily activities. It has up-to-date information, the stored data is more legitimate, accurate and reliable; and the tools that accompany it reduce the possibility of error (CANÊO, 2014).

The implementation of the e-SUS Sistema Atença Bàsica (E-SUS AB), makes computerized management of Basic Health Units (UBS) possible. The software is available from the Ministry of Health at http://dab.saude.gov.br/portaldab/esus. The aim is to provide connectivity to more than 13,000 UBS, in a partnership between the Ministries of Health and Communications. e-SUS AB makes it possible to implement the Electronic Citizen's Record, which contains the user's record of care, as well as management solutions, such as controlling the stock of medicines and supplies, scheduling appointments and monitoring the workload of professionals (as described on the SUS portal for primary care). eSUS Atençao Bàsica (e-SUS AB) is a strategy of the Department of Primary Care (DAB) to restructure primary care information at national level. This action is in line with the more general proposal to restructure the Ministry of Health's Health Information Systems, understanding that the qualification of information management is fundamental to improving the quality of care provided to the population. The e-SUS strategy refers to the process of qualified computerization of the SUS in search of an electronic SUS (BRASIL, 2014).

E-SUS AB has become a highly resolutive technological tool, as it gathers all the information needed for progressive user care in real time, avoiding repetitive procedures. Its contribution is not limited to retrieving information about the user, but also to integrating the billing and cost calculation areas; it has provided electronic medication checks for the nursing team, in accordance with the opinion issued by the Federal Nursing Council (COFEN); allowed compliance with the Resolution of the Federal Council of Medicine (CFM) which provides for the legibility of every medical act prescribed; guaranteed the mapping of consultations carried out by each professional and contributed to administrative analysis of the time spent on user care by each of those who work there (CANEO, 2012).

In the municipality of Fortaleza, Ceará, Brazil, the primary health care units have been computerized, keeping them interconnected. In 2002, the health units had microcomputers in practically every room. Registration, scheduling, referrals, prescriptions, dispensing of medicines, requesting tests, viewing tests, management reports and recording consultations were all computerized. Around 82 units were interconnected at the time of implementation. A medical record registered at one unit could be accessed at any other point. Implementation took place gradually, with mobilization involving providers (doctors, nurses, etc.) and the public. In 2005, the new municipal administration reviewed the contract and decided to terminate it. As of March 2006, the system could no longer be updated, as the municipality did not own the rights to the program. The contract was terminated in 2005, and a new system was launched in 2007, and then re-implemented in 2009 (HOLANDA, 2008).

The health sector has benefited from the use of information technology, especially in the use of demographic and health information systems, which are of fundamental importance for the practice of surveillance and monitoring of diseases and indicators of morbidity and mortality (CLOCK, 2014).

TAT presents an alternative for promoting the health of hypertensive patients with the use of Information and Communication Technologies (ICT), through *software that is* applicable because health professionals are increasingly using resources such as computers and cell phones to speed up user care.

[...] *the application of the TAT is interesting, but the unit needs to be better organized, because it increases the consultation time and the user usually doesn't want to wait long* [...] (E37)

Accessibility allows people to get to the health institution and experience the correct use of services in order to achieve the best possible results. In this case, it includes aspects of the organization and dynamics of these institutions.

[...] *the TAT is applicable as long as the professionals have the necessary consultation time to evaluate the patients* [...] *also when we have enough teams so as not to overload the professional* [...] (M49, M56)

[...] *unfeasible, large number of items, we have little time for the patient* [...] *the questionnaire is very long, it is unfeasible to fill it out given our daily demand for care, which is affected by the lack of staff* [...] (E32, E88, M102)

It involves strategic planning, which is a set of items within an organization that need to be researched, analyzed and outlined in order to achieve objectives and goals. It is a very efficient tool, especially when there is integration between those who manage and those who carry out the actions. In a world where things change, where what was known yesterday is no *longer* exactly useful today, organizations need people who think. It doesn't involve future decisions, but the future implications of present decisions (SILVA, 2014).

According to Penchansky and Thomas *apud* Travassos and Martins (2004), access consists of five dimensions: *welcoming* - which represents the relationship between the way services are organized to receive users and the ability of these users to adapt to this organization; *accessibility* - characterized by the adequacy between the geographical distribution of services and users; *acceptability* - represents the attitudes of users and health professionals towards each other's characteristics and practices; *availability* - volume and types of services in relation to user needs; and *purchasing capacity* - defined by the relationship between ways of financing services and people's ability to pay for these services.

The condition cited by the professional for the applicability of the TAT refers directly to the availability of human resources adequate to the demand of users, both in terms of the number of EqSF and the diversity of professional categories, prioritizing the establishment of a link with the EqSF, avoiding the rotation of professionals in user care.

The 5 (13.6%) FHTs who opposed the feasibility and applicability of the TAT justified their position on the grounds of the time stipulated per consultation, the length of the instrument, the unavailability of the user with the waiting time for the consultation, and the deficit in the number of FHTs.

[...] *with the time stipulated at 15 minutes per visit, a very dense evaluation instrument can compromise the consultation* [...] for the *current reality of care in health units, the instrument is extensive to be filled out during consultations* [...] (E6, M46)

The TAT, in its entirety, involves all the data that should be included in a consultation: identification data; anamnesis data, when assessing CCH; and physical examination and laboratory findings when assessing IAT. Therefore, in the case of a consultation with a hypertensive user, the TAT does not prolong time, but rather facilitates the clinical assessment procedure, treatment follow-up, therapeutic decision-making and the provision of educational guidance. Therefore, the application of the TAT in conjunction with the EqSF consultation will complement integrated care for hypertensive clients.

[...] *TAT is excellent* [...] *however, it takes a long time to perform and patients are usually very stressed and don't like to wait* [...] (M38)

The justification for refusing to apply the TAT refers to reception, which represents the relationship between the way services are organized to receive users and the ability of these users to adapt to this organization. We agree with Fertig (2014) in highlighting the importance of humanizing the process of welcoming users, in which diversity must be respected and subjectivities deserve a more accurate look, with a better understanding of all the problems that affect those who seek health services. The principles and guidelines of the Unified Health System (SUS) reveal a proposal for humanization and welcoming. It is necessary to promote reflection on the practices of health professionals working in health services. The perception that users can develop with the welcoming service is that they will be cared for at the USF and not referred to another service. This is related to the resoluteness and resolution of the user's demands.

Nine (90.0%) judges admitted the viability and applicability of the TAT, regardless of the type of institution - public or private.

[...] *the proposed TAT is totally feasible and of excellent applicability, being an important tool for measuring hypertensive patients' adherence to treatment, in both public and private services* [...] (J3, J4, J6, J7, J9)

There is still no effective and efficient instrument or technology for assessing adherence to treatment, although there are around 12 (twelve) instruments available in the literature. However, each of these tools has a shortcoming that makes it unfeasible in care practice. However, the shortcoming that is common to all of them is that they only assess drug treatment. Therefore, there is no gold standard instrument for assessing adherence.

According to Franco (2013) and Leandro (2013), to date, self-reporting, pill counting, electronic packaging, prescription renewals in closed pharmacy systems and serum drug levels have been used. According to Leandro (2013), direct methods involve measuring the serum level of the drug, are expensive and are not universally available. They have restricted access and are generally found in research laboratories, which contributes to the high use of indirect methods, which are simpler and lower cost, useful for clinical practice and can provide valuable information. According to Santa Helena (2008), instruments that take self-reporting into account are generally based on an epidemiological approach where the evaluation should be as accurate as possible. Most self-report questionnaires are more feasible, but have low sensitivity and high specificity (SANTA HELENA, 2008).

Only one (10.0%) judge was against the feasibility/applicability of the TAT, particularly in the item referring to the "appropriate use of salt", focusing on the exact measure of salt to be consumed by the hypertensive person.

[...] *I found the applicability difficult for the EqSF, very subjective. For example: in the proper use of salt, does the doctor know what the amount of sodium corresponds to?* (J5)

Health professionals who conduct themselves in accordance with the guidelines know perfectly well how much sodium a hypertensive individual should use. There are individual differences in sensitivity and even modest reductions in the amount of salt are generally effective in reducing BP. This evidence reinforces the need to advise hypertensive and "borderline" individuals on the benefits of reducing sodium in their diet. The nutritional requirement for sodium in humans is 500 mg (about 1.2 g of salt). The WHO establishes 5 g of sodium chloride or table salt (which corresponds to 2 g of sodium) as the maximum healthy daily intake (NAKASATO, 2004).

In care practice, the amount of salt consumed by hypertensive people is assessed through taste, since culturally they are used to consuming foods with a high sodium content, so their taste buds are less sensitive to this substance. Therefore, the hypertensive person is consuming the right amount of salt when they do not perceive its taste in the food, i.e. they perceive that salt has not been added.

Aspects inherent in SAH treatment modalities

The EqSF (100.0%) and the judges (100.0%) stated that the TAT satisfactorily meets the treatment modalities for SAH.

The *guidelines* reinforce that there are two types of treatment for hypertension: non-pharmacological (or hygiene measures) and pharmacological. Hygienic measures or lifestyle changes are of great importance, but they should never delay pharmacological treatment, according to risk stratification, and will always be continuously linked to drug treatment.

Aspects inherent in adherence to SAH treatment

For 99 (90.0 %) FHTs, the TAT covers all the aspects inherent in hypertensive users' adherence to treatment, because it covers the items that make up both modalities.

It is based on the current Brazilian guidelines for the control of hypertension and up-to-date literature, and presents complete and accessible content.

[...] *TAT includes both drug and non-drug treatment [...] from the assessment of diet and habits, including the approach to licit and illicit drugs, in short, it includes all the procedures that are necessary to achieve control of hypertension* [...] (E8, M12, M60)

[...] *as a light technology, the TAT will help a lot in clinical management, assisting the professional. The TAT is well structured and satisfactory for guiding care, including helping to stratify patients' risk, as well as the risks of cardiovascular complications [...]* it *is well based on the latest consensuses, guidelines and up-to-date literature* [...] (E17, E22, M99, E106)

As mentioned above, the *guidelines* consider the importance of the two treatment modalities - non-pharmacological and pharmacological, which are well grounded in TAT. However, the treatment modality routinely focused on is medication, and hygiene measures are neglected in relation to their importance.

Hygiene measures are fundamental and can be equivalent to monotherapy with drugs. However, they have a low level of adherence over time. With the level of agreement of the survey participants, there is a consensus that they can delay or prevent hypertension in non-hypertensive patients. They can prolong or avoid drug treatment in Stage I hypertensive patients and help reduce BP in hypertensive patients belonging to other stages of classification (FRISOLI, 2011).

User care must be comprehensive. The Brazilian Constitution (Art. 198, 1988) prioritizes "comprehensive care" for preventive activities in the intervention of diseases and their complications, without prejudice to assistance services. Comprehensiveness is not just a SUS guideline. It is a set of notions relating to comprehensive care, with the coordination of professionals' actions, with a comprehensive view of the human being endowed with feelings, desires, afflictions and rationalities. ter. A coordinated team effort is needed to produce and promote care for the benefit of users, establishing links, procedures and prioritizing their needs, which will help to meet their needs and satisfy them with the service.

Health professionals who deal with hypertensive patients must seek care that goes beyond the biological level and consolidate actions that seek comprehensive and humanized care (SANTOS, 2013).

The other FHTs (10.0%) stated that the TAT has gaps related to the inclusion of hypertensive medication, and socioeconomic, religious and cultural data.

[...] *lack of use of medications that interfere with pressure: NSAIDs, corticosteroids* [...] (M50) [...] *lack of socioeconomic, religious and cultural aspects that interfere with adherence* [...] (E66, E95, E96)

Non-steroidal anti-inflammatory drugs are common causes of uncontrolled BP. They raise BP by inhibiting renal prostaglandins, with a drop in renal flow followed by fluid retention. It also interferes with other antihypertensive drugs, with the exception of calcium antagonists. The effect is more pronounced in patients with reduced renal function. Selective cyclooxygenase-2 inhibitors have similar effects. Sympathomimetic agents such as nasal decongestants, appetite control pills, cocaine and amphetamine-like stimulants, oral contraceptives, glucocorticoids, anabolic steroids and cyclosporine are also commonly used agents that interfere with BP control. Herbal supplements such as ma huang and ginseng also raise BP. The effect of these agents varies. Some patients have no change in BP while others have a severe rise. Illicit drugs can also raise BP, causing resistant hypertension (SARAFIDIS, 2008).

The use of oral contraceptives (OC) is associated with some increases in BP and the onset of hypertension in 5.0% of users. However, studies have evaluated older generation OCs, which contain a higher amount of estrogens. There is an increased risk of acute myocardial infarction (AMI) in women who use OC, particularly those who smoke. They have a 2 (two) times greater risk of stroke. The likelihood of BP rising with menopausal hormone replacement therapy is reduced. They should not be used for primary or secondary prevention of CVD. It is used to relieve severe menopausal symptoms, and the risks must be weighed against the benefits.

Socio-economic, religious and cultural data are included in the Identification of Hypertensive Users (IUH).

Eight (80.0%) judges stated that the TAT provides a perfect response to the aspects inherent in adherence to SAH treatment.

[...] *the aspects inherent to adherence are completely covered, from the clinical side to a healthy lifestyle* [...] (J3, J5)

[...] *the items are complete, covering the important aspects inherent to the treatment* [...] it *covers risk factors related to lifestyle habits, in addition to the therapy used and the systematic monitoring of BP* [...] (J6, J8)

When it comes to healthy lifestyles, you must first get to know hypertensive patients' lifestyles, routines and habits, which is extremely important for providing individualized care and proposing health interventions that take their needs and peculiarities into account. Adherence to treatment is a complex process and a challenge for patients and professionals, and the effective work of a multidisciplinary health team is important. Constant intervention strategies must be developed, encouraging people to make lifestyle changes and receive appropriate treatment. The components of a healthy lifestyle are: proper, healthy eating, physical activity, preventive awareness, interpersonal relationships, stress management and abstention from addictions. By maintaining this lifestyle, you can maintain effective control of hypertension and prevent its acute and chronic complications (GUEDES, 2013).

And 2 (20.0%) judges evaluated it incompletely in relation to the aspects mentioned, but the justifications given referred to the possible causes of non-adherence which will be investigated during the consultation which will take place after the TAT has been applied. This, in turn, will help the EqSf to guide the hypertensive person towards adherence to treatment.

[...] *in my opinion, there is a lack of reasons for non-adherence to drug/non-drug treatment and consultations, such as: cost of the drug, adverse events, lack of attention (forgetfulness), complex therapeutic regimens, lack of understanding of the disease or prescription, among others* [...] (J1)

The causes of non-adherence are investigated during the consultation, after the TAT has been applied, in order to plan and implement educational actions.

Factors related to non-adherence include: difficulty in accessing health services, complex medication regimen, misunderstanding of medical prescriptions, side effects of medication, lack of reception from the health service, lack of family support, health beliefs, large rotation of health professionals, lack of health education, low socioeconomic level of the user, low level of education (BRAND ÂO, 2012).

Health education is an instrument that facilitates the empowerment of humanity, contributing to the promotion of health. It is necessary to establish a relationship based on therapeutic listening, respecting users' life stories and beliefs, in order to establish actions through the collective construction of knowledge and practices, since an individual's health profile is related to their living conditions, the social environment in which they live, income distribution, level of education, work and leisure. An integral action based on the principles of citizenship. Educational actions are tools for exchanging popular and scientific knowledge, used to train the community in self-care and coping with the health-disease process (CERVERA, 2011).

[...] *I think it's important to ask about the undesirable effects of antihypertensive drugs, which can interfere with adherence to treatment* [...] (J9)

Several factors can influence adherence to treatment: those related to the hypertensive person (gender, age, ethnicity, marital status, schooling and socioeconomic level); to the disease (chronicity, absence of symptoms and complications); to health beliefs, lifestyle and cultural habits (perception of the seriousness of the problem, lack of knowledge, experience with the disease in the family context and self-esteem); treatment, involving quality of life (cost, undesirable effects, complex therapeutic regimens), the institution (health policy, access to health services, waiting time versus time to be seen); and the relationship with the health team. It can be due to the undesirable effects of anti-hypertensive drugs, financial barriers, the individual's lack of motivation to treat an asymptomatic disease, lifelong treatment, influence on quality of life, inadequate relationship with the health team, etc (GUSMÂO, 2006). In addition to these factors, there is also family involvement (SANTOS *et al,* 2007).

Modifications or additions to the TAT

According to Table 5, the EqSFs admitted the need for modifications and/or additions to the TAT, in relation to (to) (s):

- (30.9%) regarding the frequency of physical exercise, the daily amount of salt to be consumed, and the inclusion of foods rich in fiber.

[...] *I would put 3 to 5 days of physical activity per week [...]* (E43)

[...] *list processed foods and those rich in fiber* [...] *mention foods that help reduce AP* [...] (M93, E95, E101)

[...] *provide an estimate of the amount of salt to be ingested daily* [...] *clarify more about the proper use of salt in the*

GIAT [...] (E62, E79)

Physical exercise for people with hypertension should be in accordance with the following guidelines: aerobic (walking, running, cycling and swimming), moderate intensity, at least 30 minutes, and 5 to 7 days a week.

Detailed information on exercise and diet is available on the GIAT.

The diet should also include a low intake of saturated fat, as this increases the level of LDL-c (*low density lipoprotein*), which is deposited on the walls of the arteries.

It should be abundant in fruit, vegetables, low sugar consumption and skimmed milk. The 2004 INTERHEART study, carried out in 52 countries, proved this (SILVA, 2013).

- *aspects inherent to adherence to treatment* (18.2%), were pointed out by the EqSF in relation to the hypertensive person's opinion of the treatment and the difficulties encountered in adherence.

[...] *providing a space for users to express their opinions about treatment [...] and the difficulties in adhering to SAH treatment [...]* (E20, E65)

The consultation with the team is the ideal time and space for people to express their complaints, doubts, feelings, suggestions, etc. and be heard (SILVA, 2015).

- *stipulated scores* (36.4%) relating to abstaining from smoking, regular use of medication, attending appointments with the EqSF, controlled blood pressure, regular physical exercise, adequate use of salt, and control of glycemic levels (diabetics and non-diabetics).

[...] *I suggest increasing the score for smoking* [...] *the scores are discrepant in relation to the consumption of medicines, because there is very little* [...] (E6, E29)

Smoking cessation, as recommended by the VII Brazilian Hypertension Guidelines (2016), is a fundamental and priority measure in the primary and secondary prevention of cardiovascular and various other diseases. However, there is no evidence that there are any benefits for BP control. It shows an acute rise in BP, but its chronic effects are not yet well established (ESC/ESH,2013).

Smoking is an important risk factor (RF) for atherosclerotic cardiovascular disease. Smoking causes an acute increase in BP and HR (heart rate), which persists for more than 15 minutes. Quitting smoking is probably the most effective lifestyle change for the prevention of CVD, such as stroke, acute myocardial infarction and peripheral vascular disease and should always be encouraged (ESC/ESH, 2013).

The major obstacle is combating chemical dependence on nicotine. Nicotine addiction is a complex phenomenon because several variables are involved. Each individual must be assessed individually and various psychotherapeutic approaches such as cognitive-behavioral therapy are indicated (based on the fact that an internal and hidden process of cognition, such as thought, influences a person's emotions and behaviors) (ZANELATTO, 2013).

[...] *assign higher scores to: regular use of the medication regimen, attendance at appointments, controlled blood pressure* [...] *also maintain equal scores for controlled blood pressure and glycemic levels* (E55, M87)

The IATs are dependent on follow-up to the CCH, so the scores stipulated were based on the guidelines and specific literature.

[...] *there is a discrepancy in the regular use of the medication regimen, and regular physical exercise, so I suggest a higher score for the regular use of the medication regimen* [...] (E62)

Pharmacological and non-pharmacological therapies complement each other. Most of the time, drug treatment alone cannot control BP. The guidelines recommend both types of treatment. Regular aerobic exercise is a way of controlling hypertension, which is part of the non-pharmacological treatment through lifestyle changes, a fact that makes it as important as the use of medication.

- *instructional guide for the validation of the TAT* (GIAT) (21.8%), in relation to the "healthy eating" behavior.

[...] *improve the definition in practical quantities: for example: number of spoons and percentage of vegetables [...] add more data about food, because there are no nutritionists at the EqSF* [...] (E39, E58)

SAH affects millions of people worldwide and contributes significantly to a large number of deaths due to myocardial infarction, stroke and chronic kidney disease. SAH has a multicausal and multifactorial origin, with the environment exerting an influence on its genesis, since its onset is related to an inadequate lifestyle, as well as constitutional factors (gender, age, race and family history). Treatment consists primarily of transformative education, with the team working to make the client aware of the need to change their habits and lifestyle, improving their quality of life and reducing the rate of cardiovascular complications (SANTOS, 2012).

Through a multidisciplinary team made up of doctors, nurses, nutritionists, social workers, psychologists, dieticians and pharmacists, adherence to treatment will be significantly higher.

The participation of a nutritionist is essential, as hypertension is closely related to excess weight and salt intake, as excessive consumption can contribute to the establishment of resistant hypertension. Hypertensive patients should be advised to eat vegetables, low-fat dairy products, soluble dietary fiber, whole grains and proteins from plant sources, with a reduction in saturated fat and cholesterol, and fresh fruit. In the recommended Mediterranean diet, hypertensive individuals are advised to eat fish at least twice a week and 300-400g/day of fruit and vegetables (ESC/ESH,2013). With regard to fiber intake, they are classified as soluble and insoluble. Soluble fiber is found in oat bran, pectin (fruit) and gums (oats, barley and legumes: beans, chickpeas, lentils and peas). Insoluble fibers: cellulose (wheat), hemicellulose (grains) and lignin (vegetables). The recommended intake of total dietary fiber for adults is 20 to 30 g/day, 5 to 10 g of which should be soluble. The beta-glucan present in oats causes a slight reduction in BP in obese people, an effect not observed in normal-weight individuals (DBHA, 2016).

Disease-centered health practice disregards the complexity of the individual. The principles related to the SUS involve universal access to health services at all levels of care, comprehensive care, preservation of people's autonomy and equality of health care. For comprehensiveness to occur, a multi- and interdisciplinary approach is needed at all levels of health care. Therefore, the expanded clinic, which enables individualized care, corroborates the principle of integrality, where there is no fragmentation of the subject to diseases. It assumes a radical commitment to the individual. By recognizing the limitations of each professional area, it reveals the need to search for other knowledge in different areas. It is necessary to help the individual to transform themselves, seeking healthy lifestyles (FARÂO, 2011).

All of this involves strategic planning, which is a tool that seeks to understand a reality, integrating all of its aspects into a synthetic idea, allowing for interventions and actions aimed at a desired goal. Through knowledge of the biopolitical aspects prevailing in health, it must be evaluated and reoriented according to the majority social interests (KLEBA, 2011).

In order to expand the actions of the Family Health Strategy (ESF), the Family Health Support Centers (NASF) were created in 2008. They are made up of multi-professional teams that work together with ESF professionals to provide comprehensive physical and mental care to SUS users. The NASF team is generally made up of professionals such as a social worker, physical educator, physiotherapist, nutritionist, psychologist, psychiatrist, occupational therapist and other medical specialties.

An NASF should be made up of a team in which professionals from different areas of knowledge work together with the EqSF professionals, sharing and supporting health practices in the territories under the responsibility of the FH teams. This composition must be defined by the municipal managers themselves and the FH teams, based on criteria of priorities identified on the basis of local needs and the availability of professionals from each of the different occupations. The NASF is not a gateway to the system for users, but rather a support for the FH teams.

The NASF must act within some guidelines relating to PHC, namely: interdisciplinary and intersectoral action; ongoing health education for professionals and the population; development of the notion of territory; integrality, social participation, popular education; health promotion and humanization. It should be structured to prioritize shared and interdisciplinary care, with an exchange of knowledge, training and mutual responsibilities, generating experience for all the professionals involved, through a wide range of methodologies, such as the study and discussion of cases and situations, therapeutic projects, guidance and joint care, etc. It is made up of nine strategic areas, which are: child/adolescent and youth health; mental health; rehabilitation/integral health of the elderly; food and nutrition; social services; women's health; pharmaceutical care; physical activity/body practices; integrative and complementary practices (BRASIL, 2007).

According to Chart 5, the judges indicated modifications and/or additions to the guidelines for controlling SAH (40.0%), with regard to the meaning of the "appropriate use of salt".

[...] *define what the proper use of salt is, and specify how to use it* [...] (J1, J7)

- *stipulated scores* (40.0%) regarding control of glycemic levels and attendance at appointments.

[...] *in the indicators of adherence to treatment, the score for control of glycemic levels, in diabetic and non-diabetic users. If diabetic, score less than 90, and less than 80 in non-diabetics. The scores should be changed to cover the total of 100. High scores for attending appointments* [...] (J3, J5)

Blood glucose is one of the factors, apart from BP, used to stratify cardiovascular risk. The diagnosis of *diabetes mellitus* (DM) is confirmed with fasting plasma glucose above 126mg/dl in two repeated measurements and/or glycated hemoglobin (HbAlc) above 7%, and post-load above 200mg/dl. In non-diabetics, normal fasting glucose is less than or equal to 99 mg/dl and a normal glucose tolerance test. A higher weight for the scores was established for diabetic users because, when hypertensive, this category is considered to be at high or very high risk of cardiovascular events.

The biggest cause of hospital admissions for people with DM is cardiovascular disease. It has a high morbidity and mortality rate in these individuals. AMI and stroke are the main causes of death in people with DM. Atherosclerosis in these individuals occurs earlier and more frequently (LERARIO, 2008).

Stress hyperglycemia, which occurs in individuals admitted as victims of AMI with no previous history of DM, worsens their prognosis, with a higher rate of complications and mortality. It occurs due to adrenergic stimulation resulting from the stress associated with the myocardial ischemic event. It indicates lower pancreatic reserve and worse outcomes when comparing diabetic and non-diabetic ischemic people. It is present in around 25 to 50% of these people and is a marker of worse prognosis for outcomes such as heart failure (HF) and cardiogenic shock (MODENESI, 2012).

- *instructional guide for the validation of the TAT* (GIAT) (30.0%), there was an indication of the new guidelines for SAH in the elderly.

- ...] *I would cite the new guidelines for SAH in the elderly and change the term "lipid profile" to "lipid profile", because the lipid profile includes total lipid levels, which are not important in clinical practice* [...] (J2, J4)

In the 2013 European guidelines, elderly hypertensive patients with systemic BP greater than or equal to 160 mmHg are recommended to reduce their BP to 150-140 mmHg. In physically well elderly people under the age of 80, antihypertensive treatment can be considered for systemic BP values greater than or equal to 140 mmHg with a BP target below 140mmHg, if the treatment is well tolerated. With elderly people over 80 years of age, with initial systemic BP above 160 mmHg, it is recommended to reduce this BP to 150 and 140 mmHg, if they are in good physical and mental condition. In the frail elderly, treatment should be decided on the basis of monitoring its clinical effects. Continuation of treatment should be considered, if well tolerated, when a treated individual becomes octogenarian. All classes of medication can be used. In isolated systemic hypertension (ISH), diuretics and calcium antagonists are preferred (ESC/ESH, 2013).

As for the term "lipid profile", it is the most correct and the most widely used in the literature, because when an individual is assessed, a 12-hour fasting blood sample is taken to measure HDL-cholesterol, triglycerides and LDL-cholesterol is calculated using *Friedewald*'s formula (LDL-C=CT-(HDL-C-TG/5). It is not necessary to fast before measuring total cholesterol - Apo B and Apo A-1. Apo-B is not yet included in cardiovascular risk calculation algorithms, and has no predefined treatment target. It is the main apoprotein in the atherogenic particles made up of the lipoproteins LDL, IDL and VLDL. Apo-A1 is the main apoprotein in HDL. Apolipoproteins can be used as risk stratification, but they are not used as diagnostics or treatment targets.

The non-HDL cholesterol fraction is used as an estimate of the total number of atherogenic particles in plasma (VLDL+IDL+LDL) and also refers to Apo-B levels. Non-HDL cholesterol=CT-HDL-C.

The tables for lipid profile reference values for individuals over 20 years of age include: C-T, HDL-C, LDL-C, TG and non-HDL cholesterol (V DBL, 2013), and do not include total lipid dosage.

Other suggestions for building the proposed TAT

According to Chart 6, among the suggestions made by the EqSF, the following stand out: liaise with the Municipal Health Department (SMS) to implement the TAT on the electronic medical record platform, if approved (37.8%), implement the TAT as soon as possible, because everyone wins - users and EqSF (34.5%), and make explicit in the GIAT the periodicity of application of the TAT to assess adherence (21.8%).

[...] *drugs - analgesics, anti-inflammatories, corticoids, among others - also interfere with BP control, so they should be included in the GIAT list* [...] (M 12)

[...] *include in the item "stress management" the list of complementary therapies that have been regulated by SUS* [...] (E 17)

The use of complementary therapies is often more widely used. People facing the challenge of incurable diseases are attracted by the opportunity to have other possibilities of care. The search for these therapies aims to support conventional treatment and improve quality of life. Their use should not be exclusive or exclusionary, but integrative, as they are therapies that are compatible with the principles of palliative care and are related to the autonomy of the individual (CAIRES, 2014).

In 2003, Brazil launched the National Policy for Integrative and Complementary Practices (PNPIC) with the aim of meeting the guidelines and indications of various National Health Conferences and WHO recommendations. The PNPIC, in the Unified Health System (SUS), was approved in February 2006 and published in the form of Ministerial Ordinances n. 971 on May 3, 2006 and n. 1.600, of July 17, 2006 (BRASIL, 2006).

The complementary therapies used are: acupuncture, auriculture, chromotherapy, *Do-In,* herbal medicine, yoga, massage, meditation, music therapy, reflexology, *reiki, shiatsu,* dance therapy, therapeutic touch and visualization. Complementary therapies are considered to be therapies that promote the relief of physical, psychological and emotional symptoms. Music therapy is widely used. It can produce positive changes in mood, restore peace and emotional balance, enhance emotional expressiveness and promote relaxation and the expression of feelings such as sadness, anger and grief. It is also a communication resource, which can establish interpersonal relationships, help bring back feelings and memories from the past, providing well-being and comfort to the sick person and their caregivers/family members.

As mentioned above, complementary therapies are used more in palliative care but can also be a complementary therapy in many chronic diseases.

[...] *implementation of the electronic medical record through coordination with the municipal Health Department, for better evaluation of users, due to the time factor, practicality [...] because the TAT is very interesting* [...] (E32, E35)

Health technology involves knowledge that uses material and non-material resources in the production of health services. These resources are developed during work practices in primary care, and should include various technologies in an appropriate manner, according to health needs. From this perspective, technologies are characterized as the actions and health services needed to promote better conditions for users. Technologies are analyzed as light, light-hard and hard. Soft technologies are those that involve relationships such as bonding, decision-making, welcoming and organizing the work process. Soft-hard technologies are well-structured knowledge in the health work process. Hard technologies are technological equipment (machines), standards and organizational structures. It is therefore a resource of the health production process, which occurs continuously, involving knowledge, equipment and machines. As part of light technology, welcoming directs the establishment of care strategies, involving workers, managers and users. In this way, the needs felt by users can be worked on by the Family Health Program (PSF) teams in order to provide solutions to real health needs. In this sense, it is worth emphasizing that, when working with the technology of relationships during care, welcoming is one of the first actions to be taken by the whole team when receiving the user at the health unit. Health workers should welcome users by recognizing them by name and then taking an interest in the subjective aspects they present when they come to the health unit (COELHO, 2012).

This quality care is facilitated by the use of electronic medical records, which contain all the user's data. The TAT can be attached to this record, which not only makes it practical, but also simplifies data collection during the first assessment of hypertensive patients.

[...] *return with the results of the work to the units, so that the fruit of this study can help to change conducts/improve the care provided to the user* [...] (E 70)

You should be aware of the importance of disseminating research data when it can contribute to health promotion and the quality of life of individuals. The data is collected from a population with the help of professionals and/or users, and should be returned to them as a tool to help them change their lifestyles and therapy, because a great scientific discovery comes into existence not only because of the talent of its creator, but also because it is recognized and appropriated by the entire scientific community.

Science and technological innovation must be used to help solve humanity's serious problems, contributing to a society that is dignified, fair, supportive and sustainable. We are therefore seeing frequent investments and advances in new technologies these days.

Cell phones have been used in various areas of health care, for disease management and monitoring as *self-report* tools for self-management of people with SAH. It is very useful, especially during periods of difficult hypertension control or when changing or adjusting medication (BENGTSSON, 2014).

Through telemonitoring, the individual can also provide information at a pre-established time about their illness and receive guidance with the aim of greater adherence to hypertension treatment (MC-WORTHER, 2014).

Some existing *smartphone* apps are used to help individuals by reminding them to take their medication in the correct doses, teaching them to distinguish between drugs to avoid confusion and to avoid known potent drug interactions and common administration errors. They also provide guidance on how to store medicines properly and on healthy lifestyle habits (MIRA, 2014).

[...] *I hope that TAT is implemented as soon as possible, because everyone will win - users and professionals* [...] (E16)

In developed countries, non-adherence to treatment for chronic diseases hovers around 50%, and is probably higher in developing countries. Among these diseases, hypertension is asymptomatic and has an impact on the user upon diagnosis, especially with regard to the use of medication and lifestyle changes (WHO, 2003).

In Brazil, non-adherence rates are: 49% in Rio de Janeiro-RJ, 43.4% in Porto Alegre - RS, 86.3% in Sao Paulo, 25% in Sao Luiz and 36-42% in Fortaleza (BORGES, 2012).

The WHO cites that the magnitude and impact of low adherence in developing countries is even greater in view of the scarcity of health resources and inequalities of access (WHO, 2012).

Adherence to treatment is considered to be the patient's health-related behavior, more than just the act of using prescribed medication. The WHO defines it as the degree of a person's behavior when taking medication, following a diet and making lifestyle changes (LIMA, 2010).

The disease begins to interfere in the lives of people with hypertension from the moment they realize they are ill. It becomes difficult to convince them, as they are often asymptomatic, and they start to be labeled as hypertensive, implying sudden changes in pleasurable habits and permanent use of medication (BORGES, 2012).

[...] *I suggest the implementation of this technology in the public health service, that is, that it is really put into practice in primary care, really contributing to an effective improvement in the follow-up of people with SAH* [...] (E8, E45)

The TAT is really a working tool for the EqSF to promote the health of hypertensive individuals, which is in line with technological innovations and the principles of the National Policy for the Management and Evaluation of Health Technology (PNGTS).

The PNGTS approved in 2009 aims to maximize the health benefits obtained with the resources made available by the Ministry of Health (MS), ensuring that the population has access to effective and safe technologies, under conditions of equity (SILVA, 2012).

[...] *determine how often the TAT should be applied to evaluate the results* [...] (M51, E107)

It should be applied at the first consultation and its periodicity should be linked to the individual's return to medical consultations. In the 2013 European guidelines, patients with Stage 1 hypertension (E1) and E2 without RF, in which only lifestyle changes are recommended, should return for their first consultation after a few months. With 1-3FR, lifestyle changes and a return visit of several weeks, but without establishing the exact number of weeks or months. At this point, the TAT would be reapplied. The Brazilian guidelines recommend that at E1, the patient should be reassessed at 2 months, E2 at 1 month and E3 at 1 week. However, we know that SEM takes time; the individual is suddenly faced with a diagnosis of a chronic, asymptomatic pathology which implies a radical change in their behavior. Table 6 - Distribution of EqSF (n = 110) and judges (n = 10) according to suggestions that could contribute to the construction of the TAT. Fortaleza-Cearà-Brazil, 2017. n

=110

Suggestions	f	%
EqSF (Nurse and Doctor)		
Inclusion in the GIAT of the list of drugs that interfere with BP control	06	5,4
Inclusion in the GIAT, under "Stress management", of the list of therapies complementary services consolidated by SUS	08	7,3
Explanation in the GIAT of the frequency of application of the TAT to assess adherence	24	21,8
Number of consultations per professional (nurse) at GIAT and doctor) regulated by the DBHA and MS.	12	10,8
Articulation with the Municipal Health Department (SMS) for implementation of the TAT on the electronic medical record platform, if approved Return of the TAT results	42	37,8
to the UAPS, in order to help with the changeover	11	10,0
Improvements in the care provided to hypertensive patients Addition to the GIAT of a list of foods that help reduce BP (E101)	09	8,18
Implementation of TAT as soon as possible	38	34,5
Dissemination of the TAT in all services - public and private, following its approval	28	6,3
Determining the frequency of TAT application to evaluate results	31	28,2
Judges		
Improving the definition of items and quantifications for greater precision in assigning scores	01	10,0
Reduction of the score for "Participation in educational activities", as it is same as "Proper use of salt"	01	10,0
In the item "illicit drugs, if yes", record the drug and the time of use.	01	10,0
Dissemination of the TAT in all services - public and private, after its approval	07	70,0

The majority of judges (70.0%) suggested that the TAT should be disseminated and implemented in public and private health services.

[...] *the TAT can be put into practice, because it is useful, feasible and timely* [...] *the lack of adherence to treatment is just as problematic for public health as hypertension itself* [...] (J7)

SAH shows a direct and positive relationship with cardiovascular risk and despite progress in prevention and control, it is still a serious public health problem. In Brazil, it is estimated that the prevalence of SAH ranges from 22.7% to 43.9%. This contributes to 31.8% of Brazilian deaths from cardiovascular diseases (BRASIL, 2011).

Between 2000 and 2011, the number of deaths from CVD rose by 28.6% and in 2011, ischemic heart disease and cerebrovascular disease accounted for 61% of CVD deaths and are responsible for serious complications and sequelae that compromise the individual's performance in the family environment and in society. Low adherence is present in 50% of cases of decompensated hypertension, a barrier to blood pressure control (BRASIL, 2011).

Adherence is a complex behavioral process because it is influenced by the individual, the environment, health professionals and the quality of medical care provided. It encompasses the biological, psychological, socioeconomic and cultural dimensions (GOMES, 2014).

SAH is the main cause of consultation in primary care. It is a disease of increasing prevalence in the world, an important risk factor for the development of cardiovascular disease and a major global public health problem. However, its control is insufficient. Low adherence occurs in 50% of hypertensive patients, and 40-60% of hypertensive individuals do not use the prescribed medication, and in a greater proportion when it involves hygiene measures - adequate nutrition, combating sedentary lifestyles, abstaining from smoking and alcohol. Effective BP control involves behavioral changes and persistence in long-term treatment (SANTOS, 2013).

[...] *I suggest that once this proposal is approved, which I believe it will be, it can be disseminated to all services - public and private - so that the indicators of adherence to SAH treatment can be known, and especially the population that is not adhering, so that health education measures, associated with the participation of health teams, can reach this clientele* [...] (J4, J5, J6, J8)

Chronic non-communicable diseases (NCDs) involve complex and multivariable factors because they are diseases that are present in people's daily lives and cause changes in their daily lives, requiring behavioral changes. The main modifiable environmental factors of CVD are inadequate eating habits, a sedentary lifestyle and obesity, combined with lifestyle changes such as smoking cessation and controlling psycho-emotional stress. In terms of prevention, monitoring the prevalence of risk factors for CVD, especially those of a behavioral nature, allows for the implementation of more cost-effective preventive actions. In addition to primary prevention, health promotion has become a theoretical and practical alternative for tackling the wide range of factors that make up the current epidemiological picture of CVD.

Action on behavioral risk factors is the primary goal of disease prevention and health education has traditionally been used to achieve this goal. However, risk behaviors can be seen as responses to adverse living conditions and action must include the creation of favorable environments. The

Ottawa Charter, fruit of the First International Conference on Health Promotion, defines health promotion as "*the process of empowering the community to take action to improve its quality of life and health, including greater participation in the control of this process.*" Health promotion aims to ensure equal opportunities and provide the means for individuals and communities to have the opportunity to know and control the determinants of their health. Among its main fields are environments conducive to healthier choices, access to health information and education, the development of skills for healthy living, as well as the reorganization of health services. Community-based intervention programs have been introduced in different countries since the early 70s. The main aim of these programs is to reduce morbidity and mortality from CVD by reducing cardiovascular risk factors in communities, based on health education and existing community structures (RIBEIRO, 2012).

When the awareness-raising process is neglected, especially among users with a low socio-economic profile, which makes it difficult for them to access knowledge and schools, with a consequent low level of schooling, the incorrect use of medication can occur and lead to the individual not following medical prescriptions satisfactorily (SOARES *et al.*, 2011).

Initiatives such as new technologies to assess adherence to hypertension treatment should be carried out to improve the effectiveness of treatment and minimize its complications. Technologies that foster communication between hypertensive users and the health team, involving guidance, encouragement, follow-up and periodic reassessment, centered on care and information about the disease and treatment. Above all, it should involve the family as participants in ensuring that hypertensive patients adhere to treatment.

9. HEALTH PROMOTION ACTION PLAN FOR PEOPLE WITH SYSTEMIC ARTERIAL HYPERTENSION

In recent decades, in Brazil and other Latin American countries, there has been a change in the mortality profile, with a greater number of deaths due to chronic non-communicable diseases (NCDs), especially cardiovascular diseases (CVDs) and systemic arterial hypertension (SAH), especially in the population over 40 years of age. Its onset is occurring at an earlier age in children and adolescents.

In order to prevent and control CVD, it is necessary to focus on its risk factors (RF), which can be classified into modifiable and non-modifiable. The former include smoking, high blood pressure, hypercholesterolemia (high LDL-c), *diabetes mellitus (DM)*, obesity (BMI >30 kg/m^2), a sedentary lifestyle, abdominal fat, a diet low in fruit and vegetables and psychosocial stress. Among the non-modifiable factors, family history of premature CVD, age (men >45 years and women >55 years) and gender are relevant.

In Brazil, the main strategies for dealing with cardiovascular risk factors have been through the proposal of public health promotion (HP) policies at the collective level and the implementation of actions aimed at the individual, with a view to diagnosing and treating hypertension.

In addition to primary prevention, health promotion is a global approach to the risk factors that contribute to the development of CVDs. The Ottawa Charter defines it as the "process of empowering the community to act to improve its quality of life and health, with greater participation by the individual in controlling this process".

There should be environments conducive to healthier choices and the individual should have access to information, health education (HE), be able to develop healthy life skills, and health services should be organized for this purpose. Community-based programs should be created with the aim of reducing morbidity and mortality from CVD, with targets for reducing cardiovascular risk factors.

It is very important to establish campaigns on modifiable RF through the media, as well as in workplaces and schools.

The Family Health Strategy (ESF), a priority of the Ministry of Health (MS), is the ideal model for changing the reality of CVD in Brazil, as it brings individuals together through community work, helping to change their behavior and lifestyle habits.

Health actions in Primary Care (PC) involve health promotion, protection, disease prevention, diagnosis, treatment and rehabilitation through practices aimed at well-defined populations, taking into account the knowledge and culture of individuals and their conceptions of health and disease, identifying problems and defining priorities. Integrated and intersectoral actions with active community participation (RIBEIRO, 2012).

From the outset, the PH movement, based on its concepts and ideologies, has invested in the autonomy of individuals in relation to their health/disease process. This reveals the need to reorient health practices in an attempt to tackle social inequalities, stimulate community participation in health decisions and planning, and involve various segments of society.

In PHC, people are empowered to take care of themselves through educational actions that articulate the meanings of health and autonomy. In the context of primary care, health education (HE) is one of the main roles of professionals in family health teams (FHTs), but it extends to all levels of care.

The traditional model of health education was the biomedical one, which aimed to prevent diseases through individualistic actions, with behavioral changes established through the prescription of healthy behaviors that were passively received by the individual. This did not lead them to reflect on their health situation. In fact, the focus was on the individual and their reality. People's critical awareness of their life context should be developed, with interaction between the individual and the health professional. We should invest in group work, from the perspective that a collective environment facilitates the construction of knowledge, due to its potential to promote dialogue, reflection and the exchange of ideas.

Everyone, professionals and users, act as equals despite taking on different roles. The main objective is social transformation, not individual transformation. There must be communion between different cultures and knowledge, with the possibility of talking, listening, reflecting, questioning and learning from each other. Users must be made critically aware of their potential and weaknesses, encouraging their autonomy in finding solutions to health problems, both individually and collectively.

Health-promoting actions involve the correct use of medication, regular attendance at medical appointments, a balanced diet, weight control, regular physical exercise, salt control, adequate water intake, abstention from alcohol and tobacco, and management of conflicting situations. Reducing salt in the diet not only lowers BP, but also reduces mortality from strokes and left ventricular hypertrophy (LVH) (CUNHA, 2014).

Brazil's current epidemiological profile, with the predominance of NCDs, reveals that morbidity and mortality are associated with poor nutrition and an inadequate lifestyle. It is known that in addition to genetic factors, there are dietary factors in the genesis of these pathologies, requiring lifestyle changes in addition to the regular use of medication. Through a multidisciplinary approach, individuals should be advised during consultations about eating a diet free of salt, saturated fats and sugars. It's essential to set up groups of ES to provide advice on hygiene and the proper use of water and food.

The SUS faces a number of difficulties, such as people's low socio-economic status, high demand, lack of trained professionals, lack of time for professionals to guide people, as well as the inadequate physical structure of some health units, not only in primary care, but also at secondary and tertiary levels.

All professionals must be prepared to advise people on these hygiene and dietary measures, in accordance with the National Food and Nutrition Policy (PNAM), which states that the municipal health system is responsible for training its professionals to establish specific activities in the area of food and nutrition for people with chronic illnesses in a productive and effective way. Consultations should follow the guidelines on pathology, RF, forms of treatment, as well as guidance on individual and collective health activities, contributing to disease control and preventing complications.

As it is the third most important cause of disability in the world, the services in charge of caring for hypertensive individuals must be based on important management and planning fundamentals.

There is a huge social cost of RF and early morbidity and mortality, such as the cost of research and treatment; the suffering of the individual, the family, loss of productivity and early retirement.

A fundamental fact in relation to SAH is that each individual with SAH is unique and adopts a lifestyle in line with their beliefs, perceptions and knowledge. It is essential that professionals know how to recognize them, providing care aimed at meeting their needs, in order to facilitate adherence to treatment and empower the individual to self-care. It involves the perception of vulnerability or susceptibility, i.e. the subjective perception of personal risk of contracting a disease, its severity, where the individual associates the disease with the seriousness of the consequences; the benefits of its treatment, with the correct use of medication, and its positive consequences and perceived barriers, preventing the adoption of appropriate treatment. This pathology worries health professionals who deal with people affected by it, due to the possibility of complications and physical and psychological sequelae,

In addition to the high rates of individuals who do not take part in physical exercise and leisure activities, there is often an insufficient intake of fruit, vegetables and legumes, with a high prevalence of factors related to these habits such as hypertension, DM, low HDL-c levels, central obesity and excess weight, in addition to the fact that the majority have four or more simultaneous factors, highlighting the importance of intensifying actions to control comorbidities and change lifestyle.

A great deal of emphasis has been placed on non-pharmacological measures to control SAH, which is currently considered the first-line therapy for its control.

Among the non-pharmacological therapies, regular physical exercise stands out as an important component in improving quality of life and studies have found lower mortality and morbidity due to diseases of the cardiovascular system in physically trained individuals.

With regard to abstaining from addictions, we should mention the consumption of alcoholic beverages, such as ethanol, which, if consumed in large quantities, is capable of increasing blood pressure (BP) and the risk of cardiovascular morbidity and mortality. In addition to this addiction, smoking and the use of other illicit drugs should be avoided, as they acutely raise BP and compromise the cardiovascular system.

Another important fact is that with technological advances, people have become increasingly sedentary, leading to a higher incidence of chronic diseases. Physical exercise, on the other hand, generally shows low adherence among people with hypertension. There is a need for educational activities to encourage this practice, as it can reduce morbidity and mortality by lowering BP and associated risk factors.

Physical exercise is one of the non-medicated treatments, and has been one of the most indicated as a therapy for reducing blood pressure levels in hypertensive patients. As well as reducing these levels, it reduces the diseases caused by hypertension, cardiovascular risk factors and early death due to these complications. It can reduce RR, heart rate, improve functional capacity, cardiovascular capacity and reduce levels of anxiety and depression. It is a tool for health education, promotion and prevention. Through this non-pharmacological intervention, it is hoped to reduce risk factors, improve functional capacity, cardiovascular capacity, heart rate, as well as levels of anxiety and depression.

It is worth mentioning that the international commitment made by the country to tackle CNCDs (2011-2022), which defines among the priority actions the approach to modifiable RF (smoking, alcohol, physical inactivity, inadequate diet and obesity), represents progress (MALTA, 2011).

The factors that explain the BP-lowering effect of physical exercise can be explained by the reduction in insulin levels and the consequent reduction in renal sodium retention and basal sympathetic tone; the reduction in catecholamine levels and the release of vasodilator substances into the circulation by the skeletal muscles, among others. The regular practice of some kind of aerobic physical exercise is of great relevance to patients with borderline or stage I hypertension without other associated risk factors, who benefit from a reduction in pressure levels similar to that promoted by antihypertensive agents, without the presence of undesirable side effects.

. With regard to diet, it is difficult to follow the recommended diet due to family and social eating habits. The family is essential for proper treatment, providing emotional support for the patient. On the other hand, healthy eating habits are embedded in cultural, economic and political models, which are not always amenable to change. For this to happen, it is essential to place greater emphasis on promoting policies aimed at the determinants of these habits.

Overweight and obesity are a reality among people with SAH. In addition, most people report that they do not receive guidance or treatment to lose weight and eat a partially adequate diet. It is essential for the Family Health Strategy (FHS) team, especially the nurses, to work with SAH, using strategies that are appropriate to the socio-cultural conditions, with a view to OS and encouraging the acquisition of healthy eating habits.

Healthy eating is generally associated with normal eliminatory functions. On the other hand, healthy eating habits are embedded in cultural, economic and political models, which are not always amenable to change. For this to happen, a greater emphasis on promoting policies aimed at the determinants of these habits is essential.

Knowledge about the severity of the disease and the perception of their susceptibility motivate the individual to act, generating changes. After all, these factors together make the person aware of their proximity to other illnesses resulting from the underlying disease and lifestyle changes.

In relation to stress, there is the psychological dimension, a set of external forces that produce transitory or permanent effects on the person, and the biological dimension, which involves everything from aspects of the central nervous system to its vegetative, endocrine, immune and behavioral repercussions in general. The events that trigger it and how these circumstances interact between the individual and the environment must be assessed. In reality, the demands of a situation exceed the perceived ability to cope with it. There is an overload beyond the person's adaptive capacity, contributing to the development of organic and psychological illnesses. We mustn't forget that leisure and restful sleep are factors that contribute greatly to stress management.

Noradrenaline and adrenaline, also known as catecholamines, are responsible for most of the immediate responses to stress, such as: tachycardia, increased BP, muscle vasodilation, vasoconstriction of the digestive tract, increased bronchial caliber, hyperglycemia due to glycogenolysis, hypertriglyceridemia due to lipolysis, increased thermogenesis, piloerection, etc.

Stress is a complex psychophysiological reaction that triggers the body's need to manifest itself in the face of something that threatens its homeostasis. It is therefore a process in which the body responds to everyday events that lead the individual to adapt or not, constantly challenging its threshold to adjust to a new equilibrium.

Emotions such as anxiety, when blocked, can, by acting on the autonomic nervous system, trigger the hypertensive crisis in certain people with a genetic predisposition. Repetitive stress or an exacerbated stress response is a sign of the activation of this system. Sympathetic activity in hypertension is involved in the rate of cardiovascular morbidity and mortality.

The long-term influence of lifestyle, behavior and work-related stress on BP in men and women points to the need for changes in individual behavior and a pleasant environment in the workplace, which can have a beneficial influence on BP variation. Controlling emotional stress helps to control hypertension and other associated pathologies, as well as improving adherence to antihypertensive treatment.

It reinforces the need for clinical interventions according to cardiovascular risk and effective public policies at the population level, with a multidisciplinary and intersectoral approach and the creation of environments that favor changes in habits.

As the individual with a chronic pathology must be assessed as a whole, it is necessary, in addition to guidance on this pathology, to regularly prevent cervical, breast, ovarian, digestive system and prostate cancer in men, with regular visits to health services, in order to improve their quality of life.

One relevant aspect is that women are more frequent visitors to health services. This leads health professionals to pay more attention to the male population.

In this respect, it can be seen that the higher percentage of SAH found among women may be related to their greater tendency towards self-care and their greater demand for health services when compared to men. The low percentage of men who seek out health services in general points to the need for greater coordination between the use of epidemiological information systems and the development, improvement and monitoring of public policies aimed at men's health. It is also important to emphasize that when it comes to married people or those living with a partner, health professionals should encourage the participation of the spouse or partner in supporting the care of this family member in the treatment of SAH, and thus encourage greater adherence.

It is also of the utmost importance that the multi-professional team identifies possible difficulties related to the treatment of hypertension, since low schooling and low income can be one of the obstacles to understanding and continuing treatment. The majority of people who attend appointments are not accompanied by family members and the presence of cognitive impairment contributes to a lack of understanding of the guidelines and low adherence to treatment.

There is a lack of specific actions aimed at the elderly and at detecting problems among schoolchildren. Both groups are of great interest in relation to NCDs: the elderly, due to their biological and social vulnerability, and children and young people, due to the opportunity for early intervention, as they have shown a significant increase in obesity and sedentary lifestyles in recent years.

We must also mention the need for regular eye examinations to prevent retinopathies, especially in people with DM and SAH.

Periodic dental examinations are also recommended to prevent bacterial endocarditis, oral mucosal lesions, tooth decay and tooth loss.

Vaccinations also prevent the onset of viral and bacterial diseases, which are very common in immunocompromised individuals such as the elderly. Vaccination against influenza and pneumonia is extremely important for people with heart disease, as these infections can lead to more serious complications or decompensate the underlying disease.

We must also mention the importance of preventing hypertensive retinopathy, since the repercussions of hypertension are felt mainly in the vascular bed of target organs, including the eye, where hypertensive retinopathy (HR) is particularly prominent. Early diagnosis of signs and lesions related to RH makes it possible to assess the severity of hypertension and, above all, to monitor the progress of hypertensive organic lesions, which can lead to a reduction in visual acuity. Monitoring can be carried out through ophthalmic examinations. Among these, fundoscopy is a practical and easy method for assessing damage to target organs, as well as providing information on the activity and time of development of hypertension. Being aware of the usefulness of these tests is yet another way for clinicians to better monitor and treat the condition. Black people, hypertensive patients with uncontrolled BP, and those over 60 are at greater risk of developing RH.

Diabetic retinopathy (DR) occurs as a microvascular complication of *DM,* affecting half of all people with the condition. It is generally related to the time the disease takes to develop, glycemic control and the presence of associated diabetic nephropathy. It is a serious public health problem and requires a multidisciplinary approach to control.

10. FINAL CONSIDERATIONS

After analyzing the contributions of the professionals from the Family Health Team (nurses and doctors) and the Judges to the process of validating the TAT, it can be seen that this technology is valid, as well as feasible and applicable, due to the consensus of these participants on its structure and composition; feasibility and applicability, including the recommendation that it be implemented in public and private services that care for hypertensive users; that it guide the team in caring for hypertensive people and in health education actions, making it easier for these people to adhere to SAH treatment.

The validation of the TAT rescued the experiences of the professionals, bringing out the power of creativity, expressiveness and, above all, persistence, through the scenario of health education, which is the focus of transformations that empower people in the search for health promotion and quality of life. Therefore, the use of TAT in the monitoring of hypertensive people will enable them to engage in self-care, consequently adhering to treatment, promoting their health and achieving quality of life; resulting in a reduction in morbidity and mortality from cardiovascular disease caused by SAH, which has been the main risk factor.

This is a technology that brings great benefits to health, as there is nothing of this size in the literature. However, it must be applied and criticized, as it is not a finished product. It can serve as a source for health indicators and their monitoring. This study is not exhausted, as it is an emerging and worrying issue for public health.

In carrying out this study, the main difficulty encountered was related to the demand and cooperation of professionals to take part in the survey, as well as the time it took to return the completed questionnaires, which had to be tripled over the time initially agreed upon, making it clear that there is a need to make professionals and managers aware of the importance of the feedback that this survey can bring to the health service.

One limitation is the fact that the judges were only doctors, leaving out the nurse's contribution, which is of fundamental importance as both are responsible for systematically monitoring hypertension.

As a researcher and health professional, I recommend that the TAT be used in the first consultation and in the control consultations of users with hypertension, as it guides the behavior of professionals and directs them to adopt a healthy lifestyle, compatible with the control of hypertension and the prevention of complications resulting from this condition.

The aim of this research is to make the TAT available for incorporation into primary care, as an essential tool for the Family Health Team in monitoring hypertensive users. It is worth pointing out that the results of this study could enable managers and the Family Health Team (FHT) to (re)plan strategies, with the aim of expanding actions to ensure that hypertensive users adhere to treatment, strengthening the basic principles of the Unified Health System (SUS) - universality, equity and comprehensiveness, promoting their health and that of their families, Consequently, minimizing the problem of hypertension for public health, which will increase with the predominance of elderly people in the Brazilian population, predicted for 2020, which will probably lead to an increase in the prevalence of this condition, since it rises with age, if all possible efforts are not implemented for its early detection and control, since it has been a major risk factor for cardiovascular and cerebrovascular diseases.

11. REFERENCES

AKKINA, SK; *et al.* Illicit drug use, hypertension, and chronic kidney disease in the US adult population. **Trans L Res,** 160 (6);391-8, 2012 Dec .

AMERICAN DIABETES ASSOCIATION (ADA, 2013), **Diabetes care,** VOl 36, suppl, January, 2013.

CAUTER, EV Sleep disturbances and insulin resistance. **Diabetes med.** 28,1455-1462 (2011).

ESH/ESC Guidelines for the management of arterial hypertension. **Journal of Hypertension** , v.31, n.7, p. 1281-1357, July 2013.

SANTOS, ZMS A; SILVA, RM **Modelo de educaçao em saùde para o selfcuidado.** Fortaleza: Universidade de Fortaleza: UNIFOR, 2002.

BRAZILIAN SOCIETY OF CARDIOLOGY. V Diretriz Brasileira de Dislipidemias e Prevençao da Aterosclerose. 2013. **Arq Bras Cardio** l. 2013;101 (4 Suppl.1) :1-22.

BRAZILIAN SOCIETY OF CARDIOLOGY. VII Diretrizes Brasileiras de Hipertensao Arterial Sociedade Brasileira de Cardiology. Sociedade Brasileira de Hypertension; 2016. **Arch**

Bras Cardiol 2010;95(1(Suppl.1):1-51).

World Health Organization (WHO). **Adherence to long-term therapies** : evidence for action. Geneva (Switzerland); 2003.

COSTA, GM, DEBS, PG, DE LA NOVAL, GR, DUENAS, HA Conocimientos, creencias y practicas en pacientes hypertensos, relacionados con su adherencia therapeutica. **Rev Cuba Enferm** , Habana, v. 21, n. 3, p. 1-1, 2005.

AKKINA, SK, RICARDO, AC, PATEL, A., DAS, A., BAZZANO, LA, BRECKLIN, C.

Illicit drug use, hypertension, and chronic kidney disease in the US adult population. **Trans L Res,** 160 (6);391-8, 2012 Dec .

ALFONSO, LM; VEA, HDB; ABALO, JA G. Validation of the MBG (Martin-Bayarre-Grau) questionnaire to assess therapeutic adherence in arterial hypertension **. Rev Cubana Salud Pùblica** , Habana, v. 34, n. 1, Jan.-Mar. 2008.

ALHALAIQA, F., DEANEE, KHO, NNAWAFLEH, AH, CLARK, A., GRAY, R. Adherence therapy for medication non-compliant patients with hypertension: a randomized controlled trial. **Journal of human hypertension** , v. 26, n. 2, p. 117-126, 2012.

ALMEIDA, PF; GIOVANELLA, L. Avaliaçao em Atençao Bàsica à Saùde no Brasil: mapeamento e anàlise das pesquisas realesados e/ou financiadas pelo Ministério da Saùde entre os anos de 2000 e 2006. **Cad Saude Publica** , v. 24, n. 8, p. 1727 -42, 2008.

BATALLA, MC., BLANQUER,A.,CIURANA,R.,GARCIA,M.,CASES,E.,PÉREZ,A. Compliance with pharmacological prescription in hypertensive patients. **Aten Primaria** , v. 1, n. 4, p.185-191, 1984.

BEN, A. J.; NEUMANN, CR; MENGUE , S.S. Morisky-Green tests and Brief Medication Questionnaire to frequently evaluate medications . **Rev Saude Publica** , Sao Paulo, v. 46, n. 2, abr. 2012.

BENGTSSON, Ulrika *et al* . Developing an interactive mobile phone self-report system for self-management of hypertension. Part 1: Patient and professional perspectives. **Blood pressure** , n. 0, p. 1-8, 2014.

BERKMAN, ND; SHERIDAN, SL, DONAHUE, KE, HALPERN,, DJ, CROTTY,,, K., Low health literacy and health outcomes: an updated systematic review **. Ann Intern Med.** 2011;155(2): 97-107.

BLOCH, KV; MELO, AN; NOGUEIRA, AR Prevalência da adesao ao tratamento anti-hypertensivo em hypertensos resistentes e validationaçao de très métodos indiretos de avaliaçao da adesao. **Cad Saude Publica,** Rio de Janeiro, v. 24, n.12, p. 2979-2984, dez. 2008.

BORGES, JWP *et al* . The use of validated questionnaires to measure the prevalence of arterial hypertension : an integrative review . **Revista da Escola de Enfermagem da USP** , v. 46, n. 2, p. 487-494, 2012.

BOSWORTH, BH *et al* . Two self-management interventions to improve hypertension control: a randomized trial. **Ann Intern Med** , v. 151, n. 10, p. 687-695, nov. 2009.

BRAAM, RL *et al* . Bromide as marker for drug adherence in hypertensive patients. **Br J Clin Pharmacol** , Londres, v. 65, n. 5, p. 733-736, feb. 2008.

BRANDAO, AA; AMODEO, C; NOBRE, F. **Hypertension.** 2nd ed. Rio de Janeiro: ELSEVIER, 2012.

BRAZIL, Ministério da Saùde. **National Policy of Integral Care for Home Health (principio e diretrizes) Brasilia, 2009.** Available at:

< http://portal.saude.gov.br/portal/arquivos/pdf/politica_nacional_atencao_integral.pdf >. Accessed : 04 Nov 2014.

BRAZIL, Ministério da Saùde. **Dos models, mapeamento e anâlise de atençao primárica à saùde nos paises da América do Sul, 2014.**

BRAZIL, Conselho Nacional de Saùde (BR). **Resolution n. 466/2012. Dispoe sobre diretrizes e norma reguladoras de pesquisas involving seres humanos** . Brasilia (DF): Conselho Nacional de Saùde; 2012.

BRAZIL. Ministry of Health. DATASUS 2009. Available at www.datasus.gov.br . Accessed June 2013.

BRAZIL. Ministry of Health. **Saùde Brasil 2008 : 20 anos de Sistema Ùnico de Saùde (SUS)/Ministério da Saùde** , Secretaria de Vigilância em Saùde, Departamento de Anàlise de Situaçao em Saùde, Brasilia: MS; 2009.

BRAZIL, Ministério da Saùde Executive Secretariat . **Ministério da Saùde e municipios:** juntos pelo acesso integral e de qualidade à saùde.2.ed. Brasilia-DF:Ministerio da Saùde, 2013.p.1-70.

BRAZIL. Ministry of Health. VIGITEL, **Vigilância de factori de risco e proteçâo para indicias cronicas por quérito telefonico,** Secretaria de Vigilância em Saùde. Brasilia: MS; 2012.

BRAZIL, Ministry of Health. Executive Secretary. The Undersecretariat of Planning and Budgeting. **National Health Plan** - PNS : 2012-2015. Brasilia (DF): Ministério da Saùde; 2011.

BRAZIL, Ministry of Health **. Plano de açoes stratégicas para o enfrentemento das cinémoses crónicas não transmissiveis (DCNT) no Brasil 2011-2022** . Secretary of Vigilância em Saùde. Brasilia (DF): Ministério da Saùde; 2011.

BRAZIL. Ministry of Health. Secretariat of Atençao À Saùde. Departamento de Atençao Básica.. **Politica Nacional de Atençao Básica** / Ministério da Saùde, Secretaria de Atençao à Saùde, Departamento de Atençao Básica. - 4th ed. - Brasilia: Ministério da Saùde, 2007.

BRAZIL. Ordinance n. GM/MS n. 2,510, of 19 de dezembro de 2005. **Institui Comissao para Elaboraçao da Politica de Gestao Technológica no ambito do Sistema Único de Saùde (CPGT).** 2005c.

BRAZIL. Ministry of Health; Secretariat of Health Policy , D **epartamento de Atençao Básica. Arterial hypertension. Systemic. Brasilia;** 2006. (Cadernos de Atençao Bàsica, 15). BRAZIL. 2006.

BRAZIL, 2006; **The national policy of science, technology and innovation in health.** 2nd ed. Brasilia: Ministério da Saùde (Série B: Textos Básicos em Saùde).

BRAZIL. Ministry of Health (BR). **National Policy on Integrative and Complementary Practices no SUS** - PNPIC-SUS. Brasilia; 2006.

BURNIER, Michel *et al.* Measuring, analyzing, and managing drug adherence in resistant hypertension. **Hypertension** , v. 62, n. 2, p. 218-225, 2013.

BURNS, N; GROVE, SK **The practice of nursing research: appraisal, synthesis and generation of evidence.** 6th ed. St Louis-Missouri: Saunders Elsevier, 2009.

BUSS, PM Uma introduçao ao concepto de Promoçao da Saùde. In: C; ZERESNIA, D.;

FREITAS, CM **Promoçao da saùde: conceitos, reflexões, tendencias.** Rio de Janeiro (RJ): Fiocruz; p.78-87, 2003.

BUTLER, CC; ROLLNICK, S. **Adesao ao tratamento médico** . London: Mosby, 2003.

CAIRES, JS *et al.* A UTILIZAÇÂO DAS TERAPIAS COMPLEMENTARES NOS CUIDADOS PALATITIVOS: BENEFICIOS E FINALITOS. **Cogitare Enfermagem** , v. 19, n. 3, 2014.

CANÊO, P. K.; RONDINA, JM Prontuàrio Eletrônico do Paciente: conechendo as experiencias de sua implantaçao. **Journal of Health Informatics** , v. 6, n. 2, 2014.

CANESQUI, AM *et al.* **Olhares Socioanthropológicos sobre os adoecidos crônicos.** Sao Paulo: Hucitec; year 2007.

CARVALHO, ALM *et al.* Adesao ao tratamento medicamentoso em usuarios cadastrados no Programa hiperdia no municipio de Teresina (PI). **Cienc Saude Coletiva** , Rio de Janeiro, v. 17, n. 7, p. 1885-1892, 2012.

CAUTER, EV Sleep disturbances and insulin resistance. **Diabetes med.** 28,1455-1462 (2011).

WAX. SECRET ARIA DO ESTADO DE SAÙDE DO CEARA - SESA. **Inform Epidemiological Doenças Crônicas Nao Transmissiveis.** p.1-6. Aug. 2013

WAX. SECRETARIA DO ESTADO DE SAÙDE DO CEARA - SESA. **Inform Epidemiology - Systemic Arterial Hypertension** . Feb. 2012.

CERVERA, DPP; PARREIRA, BDM; GOULART, BF Educaçao em saùde: percepçao dos enfermeiros da atençao básica em Uberaba (MG). **Ciênc saùde coletiva** , v. 16, n. S1, p. 1547-54, 2011.

CLOCK, D *et al.* *UTILIZATION OF* INFORMATICS RESOURCE NA SAÙDE - DIDACTIC PRACTICE IT 'S AROIO MATERIAL . **Colòquio Internacional de Educaçao e Seminàrio de Estratégias e Açoes Multidisciplinares** , v. 2, n. 1, p. 1011-1024, 2014.

COELHO, M. O; JORGE, MS B; DE ARAÙJO, ME O acesso por meio do acolhimento na atençao básica à saùde. **Revista Baiana de Saùde Pùblica** , v. 33, n. 3, 2012.

COOK, N.R .; CUTLER, JA .; *et al* . Long-term effects of dietary sodium reduction on cardiovascular disease outcomes: observational follow-up of the trials of hypertension prevention (TOHP). **BMJ,** 2007;334:885-888.

COSTA, R.S.; NOGUEIRA, LT Contributuiçao familiar no controle da hypertensao arterial. **Revista Latino-Americana de Enfermagem** , v. 16, n. 5, p. 871-876, 2008.

CUNHA, Alessandra Flores yes; et al. O AUTOCUIDADO DO ADULTO

HYPERTENSION. **Revista Interdisciplinar de Estudos em Saùde** , v. 3, n. 2, p. 55-71, 2014.

DIMATTEO, MR Variations in patient adherence to medical recommendations: a quantitative review of 50 years of research. **Med Care** , California, v. 42, n. 3, p. 200-209, mar. 2004.

DOSSE, C. et al. Factors associated to patients' noncompliance with hypertension treatment. **Latin-American Journal of Nursing** , v. 17, n. 2, p. 201-206, 2009.

DOURADO, C. S. et al. Adesao ao tratamento de idosos com hypertensao em uma unidade básica de saùde de Joao Pessoa, Estado da Paraiba. **Acta Scientiarum: Health Sciences** , v. 33, n. 1, 2011.

ESH/ESC Guidelines for the management of arterial hypertension. **Journal of Hypertension** , v.31, n.7, p. 1281-1357, ul. 2013.

Evidence-Based Guideline for the Management of High Blood Pressure in Adults Report From the Panel Members Appointed to the Eighth Joint National Committee FAJARDO, Carolina. The importance of neo-pharmacological approach to arterial hypertensive disorders in primary health care . **Revista Brasileira de Medicina de Familia e Comunidade** , [SI], v. 1, n. 4, p. 107-118, Nov. 2010.

ESTEVAN, M. C. *et al.* Estratégias de intervençao para adesao ao tratamendo da hypertensao arterial. **Ciência, Cuidado e Saùde** , v. 7, 2013.

FARAO, E. M. D. *et al* . EXTENDED CLINIC EM UM UNIVERSITY HOSPITAL: Abrindo Caminhos Para Uma Nova Forma de Cuidar. **Contexto & Saùde magazine** , v. 11, n. 20, p. 813-816, 2013.

FERTIG, A; BRAGA, FS; WITT, RR A PERCEPÇÂO DO USUARIO DA ATENÇÂO PRIMARIA SOBRE O ACOLHIMENTO EM UNIDADE DE SAÙDE DA FAMILIA. **Revista de Enfermagem** , v. 9, n. 9, p. 1-13, 2014.

FRISOLI, TM; SCHIMIEDER, RE; GRODZICKI, T.; MESSERLI, FH; Beyond salt: lifestyle modifications and blood pressure. **European heart journal** , p. Ehr379, 2011.

FOSCAL, S.; UDES, B.; UNIVERSITY, Fundación Favaloro. Consenso latino americano de hypertensao em pacientes com diabetes tipo 2 e syndrome metabolica. **Arq Bras Endocrinol**

Metab , v. 58, p. 3, 2014.

FRANCO, FGM ET al. Challenges and Solutions for Lack of Adherence to Orientations and Treatments. **Rev Soc Cardiol Estado de Sao Paulo,** v. 23, n° 2, Apr-Jun, 2013.

GARBER, M. C. The concordance of self-report with others measures of medication adherence: a summary of the literature. **Med Care** , California, v. 42, n. 7, p. 649-652, 2004.

GIACOMIN, Karla Cristina. Relatório do Conselho Nacional do Idoso Gestao 2010 2012. **Revista Portal de Divulgaçao** , n. 30, 2013.

GIROTTO, Edmarlon *et al.* Adesao ao tratamento pharmacologico e nao pharmacologico e factori associados na atençao primary da hypertensao arterial. **Ciência Saùde Coletiva** , v. 18, n. 6, p. 1763-72, 2013.

GOMES, A. *et al* . Adesao ao tratamento clinico ambulatory da systemic arterial hypertensao . **Acta Paulista de Enfermagem** , v. 27, n. 3, p. 266-272, 2014. salt: lifestyle modifications and blood pressure. **Eur Heart Journal** 2011;32:3081-30876.

GUEDES, D. et al. Hyperdia: planning and methods. **Ciência & Consciência** , v. 1, 2008.

GUEDES, NG et al. Revisao do diagnosiso de enfermagem Estilo de Vida Sedentàrio em pessoas com hypertensao arterial: conceitual analysis . **Revista da Escola de Enfermagem da USP** , v. 47, n. 3, p. 742-749, 2013.

GUSMAO JL, GINANI, GF, SILVA GV, ORTEGA, KC,. Adesao ao tratamento em isolated systolic arterial hypertension . **rev. Bras Hipertens** , v.16, n.1, p. 38-43, 2009

GUSMAO, JL; MION JR, D.; Adesao ao tratamento-conceitos. **Rev Bras hypertens** v.13: 23-25, 2006.

HALPERN, MT *et al* . Recommendations for evaluating compliance and persistence with Hypertension Therapy using retrospective data. **Hypertension** , Dallas, v. 47, p.1039-1048, Jun. 2006. Available at: < http://hyper.ahajournals.org/content/47/6/1039>. Access em: 05 Jul. 2013.

HAMILTON, GA **.** Measuring adherence in hypertension clinical trial. **Eur J Cardiovasc Nurs** , Amsterdam, v. 2, n. 3, p. 219-228, June, 2003.

HAYNES, RB et al. Can simple clinical measurements detect patient noncompliance? **Hypertension** , Dallas, v. 2, n. 6, pp. 757-764, Nov./Dec. 1980. Available at: < http://hyper.ahajournals.org/content/2/6/757 >. Acessso em: 05 Jul. 2013.

HELENA, ETS; NEMES, MIBN; Neto, JE Desenvolvimento e validaçao de questionàrio multidimensional para medir nao-adesao ao tratamento com medicamentos. **Rev Saude Publica** ,

Sao Paulo, v. 42, n. 4, p. 764-767, 2008.

HELENA, ETS; GERMAN, MIB; ELUF-NETO, J. Valiaçao da assistance a pessoas com hypertensao arterial em Unidades de Estratégia Saùde da Familia. **Saùde e Sociedade** , v. 19, n. 3, 2010.

HOLANDA, AA **Prontuàrio eletrònico do paciente** : uso, aceitaçao por médicos da atençao primárica. Fortaleza, 2008. 77 p. Dissertaçao (Mestrado em Saùde Collective).

Universidade de fortaleza, UNIFOR.

HOLT, EW *et. of* Health-related quality of life and antihypertensive medication adherence among older adults. **Age and Aging** , n. 39, p. 481-487, May 2010. Available at: http://ageing.oxfordjournals.org/ by guest on December 4, 2012 Accessed on : June 12, 2013.

ISKANDAR, JI **Normas da ABNT commented for scientific works.** 5th ed. **Curitiba: Juruà, 2012.**

JARDIM, Paulo César B. Veiga *et al.* High blood pressure and some risk factors in a Brazilian capital. **Arquivos brasileiros de cardiologia** , v. 88, n. 4, p. 452-457, 2007.

(JNC 8). **Jam.** 2014;311(5):507-520. doi:10.1001/jama.2013.284427 Published online December 18, 2013.

KAVEY, RA et al. American Heart Association Guidelines for Primary Prevention of Atherosclerotic Cardiovascular Disease Beginning in Childhood. **Circulation 2003;107:1562-66.**

KLEBA, ME; KRAUSER, IM; VENDRUSCOLO, C. A situational strategic planning no ensino da gestao em saùde da familia. **Texto and Contexto Enfermagem** , v. 20, n. 1, p. 184, 2011.

KROUSEL-WOOD, M. *et al.* New medication adherence scale versus pharmacy fill rates in hypertensive seniors. **Am J Manag Care** , v.15, n. 1, p. 59-66, Jan. 2009. Available at: < http://www.ncbi.nlm.nih.gov/pubmed/19146365 >. Accessed: 12 Jun 2013.

KIM, MT, HILL, MN, BONE, UR, LEVINE, DM Development and testing of the hill-bone compliance to high blood pressure therapy scale **. Prog Cardiovasc** Nurs. 2000;15(3):90-6

LACHAINE, Jean et al. Choices, persistence and adherence to antihypertensive agents: evidence from RAMQ data. **Canadian Journal of Cardiology** , v. 24, n. 4, p. 269-273, 2008.

LEANDRO, AW **Instrumentos de avaliaçao na adesâo do usuàrio ao tratamento da hypertensao arterial-uma systematica revisao** . Dissertaçao de Masterado Universidade de Fortaleza-UNIFOR 2013.

LEOPARDI, MT **Methodology for research on health.** 2 ed. Florianópolis: UFSC/ Pósgraduaçao em Enfermagem, 2002.

LERARIO, AC; *et al.* Assessment of the prevalence of diabetes and hyperglycemia of stress, no acute myocardial infarction. **Arq Bras Endocrinol Metab** . 2008;52(3):465-472.

LIBERTAD, M.; BAYARRE, H. Therapeutic adherence and psychosocial factors in hypertensive patients. **Rev Cubana Med Gen Integr** , v. 23, n. 1, p. 1, 2007.

LIMA, HP et al. Adesao do usuàrio hypertenso ao tratamento ea interface com o saber sobre o agravo. 2010. Rev. Renee. Fortaleza, v. 11, n. 2, p. 170-178, Apr./Jun.2010 **Rev. Renee. Fortaleza** , v. 11, n. 2, p. 170-178, April/June 2010

LIMA, T. M.; MEINERS, MMM A.; SOLER, O. Perfil de adesao ao tratamento de pacientes hypertensos atendidos na Unidade Municipal de Saùde de Fâtima. Belém, Parà, Amazonia, Brazil. **Rev Pan-Amaz Saùde. [Internet]** , v. 1, n. 2, p. 113-20, 2010.

LOBIONDO-WOOD, G.; HABER, **J. Pesquisa em Enfermagem : Methods,** critical evaluation and utilization. 4 ª ed. Rio de Janeiro: Guanabara-Koogan. 2001 **.**

LYNN, MR Determination and quantification of content validity. Nursing research, v. 35, n. 6, p. 382-386, 1986., em Belém, Parà, Amazônia, Brasil. **Rev Pan-Amaz Saude** 2010; 1(2):113-120.

MACEIRA, AM et al. Long term effects of cocaine on the heart assessed by cardiovascular magnetic resonance at 3T. **Journal of Cardiovascular Magnetic Resonance** , v. 16, n. 1, p. 26, 2014.

MACHADO, CR **Prevalencia de hypertensao arterial e factori associados,** Cambé-PR, 2012. Monograph (Especializaçao em Saùde Coletiva e Saùde da familia). Centro Universitario Filadelfia. London-PR, 2012.

MALTA, D. C.; MERHY, E. M.. O percurso da linha do cuidado sob a perspectiva das diseños crónicas nao transmissiveis. **Interface (Botucatu)** , v. 14, n. 34, p. 593-605, 2010.

MALTA, DC; MORAIS NETO, OL; SILVA JUNIOR, Jarbas Barbosa yes. Apresentaçao do plano de açoes estráticas para o enfrentemento das inésociados crónicas nao transmissiveis no Brasil, 2011 a 2022. **Epidemiologia e Serviços de Saùde** , v. 20, n. 4, p. 425-438, 2011.

MANCILHA-CARVALHO, Jairo de Jesus *et al* . The Yanomami Indians in the INTERSALT study. **Arquivos brasileiros de cardiology** , v. 80, n. 3, p. 295-300, 2003.

MARI, JJ; WILLIAMS, P. A validity study of a Psychiatric Screening Questionnaire (SRQ-20) in primary care in the city of Sao Paulo **. Br J Psychiatr** , Londres, v. 148, p. 23-26, Jan. 1986.

MARQUES, I.R .; SOUZA, AR Technology and humanization in critical care environments.

Revista brasileira de enfermagem , v. 63, n. 1, p. 141-144, 2010.

MARTINEZ, MC; LATORRE, MRDO; Fatores de risco para hypertensao arterial e diabetes melito em trabajoles de empresa metalùrgica e siderùrgica . **Arq Bras Cardiol.** 2006;87:471-9

MATOS, Y.; MEDDINGS, J. *et al.* Physician assessments of medication adherence and decisions to intensify medications for patients with uncontrolled blood pressure: still no better than a coin toss. **Health Services Research** , v. 12, n. 270, p. 1-11, 2012. Available at: < http://www.biomedcentral.com/1472-6963/12/270 >. Accessed: 03 Jun 2013.

MC-WORTHER LS; *e tal ,* The Utah remote monitoring Project: improving health care one patient at a time. **DIABETES TECHNOLOGY & THERAPEUTICS** Volume 16, Number 10, 2014

MEHRY, EM ; FRANCO, TB **Reestruturaçao Produtiva e Transiçao Tecnológica na Saùde.** um olhar a partir do cartao nacional de saùde. Campinas, 2003. (Theses - Doutorado - Universidade Estadual de Campinas).

MENDES, O.; LM *et al* . FATORES ASSOCIADOS A NÂO ADESAO AO TRATAMENTO DA HYPERTENSAO ARTERIAL SISTÈMICA: UMA REVISÂO INTEGRATIVA. Univap **Magazine ,** v. 20, n. 35, p. 56-68, 2014.

MENDES, MS *et al.* Adesao do idoso ao tratamento da hypertensao arterial siatemica: an integrative review. **Cogitare Enfermagem** , v. 17, n. 1, 2012.

MENDONÇA, L. B. A; LIMA, F. E. T.; OLIVEIRA, SKP Encephalic vascular accidents as complications of arterial hypertension : quais sao os factori intervenientes?. **Escola Anna Nery Revista de Enfermagem** , v. 16, n. 2, p. 340-346, 2012.

MENDOZA-PARRA, S.; MERINO, J.M .; BARRIGA, OA Identification of predictive factors of therapeutic non-compliance in hypertensive adults of a community in the south of Chile **. Rev Panam Salud Publica** , Washington, v. 25, n. 2, p. 105-112, 2009.

MENDOZA, S. *et al.* Determining factors of therapeutic compliance in hypertensive adults. **Revista médica de Chile** , v. 134, n. 1, p. 65-71, 2006.

MIRA, JJ; *et al.* A Spanish pillbox app for elderly patients taking multiple medications: randomized controlled trial **. J Med Internet Res** . Apr 2014; 16(4): e99.

MIRANZI, SSC *et al.* The quality of life of individuals with diabetes mellitus is hypertensive accompanied by a family health team **. Texto and Contexto Enfermagem,** v. 17, n. 4, p. 672, 2008.

MODENESI, RF *et al.* Influence on prognosis and prevalence of stress hyperglycemia in a cohort of patients with acute coronary syndrome. **Revista brasileira de terapia intensiva,** v. 24, n. 4, p.

352-356, 2012.

MOLINA, T et al..Factores Asociados Al Control de La Hypertension En Personas Overes de 60 Anos En Espana. **Rev Esp Salud Publica** 2006;80:233-242.

MOREIRA, J. B. Comunicaçao: tecnologia leve para interaçao dos saberes e pràticas do cuidado-enfermeiro e usuàrios. **Monograph [Especializaçâo em Atençao Bàsica em Saùde da Familia]. Federal University of Minas Gerais** , 2010.

MORISKY, D. E.; GREEN, LW; LEVINE, D. M. Concurrent and predictive validity of a self-reported measure of medication adherence . **Medical Care** , v. 24, n. 1, p. 67-74, Jan. 1986.

MORISKY, DE et al. Predictive Validity of A Medication Adherence Measure in an outpatient setting . **J Clin Hypertens** , Greenwich , v. 10, n. 5, p. 348-354, 2008. Available at: < http://www.ncbi.nlm.nih.gov/pubmed/18453793 >. Accessed: 07 Jun 2013.

NAKASATO, M. Sal e Hypertensao. **Rev Bras Hypertension** 2004; 11: 95-97.

NASCIMENTO, DDG do; OLIVEIRA, MA de C. **Reflexoes sobre as competencias professionnels para o processo de trabalho nos Nùcleos de Apoio à Saùde da Familia** . O Mundo da Saùde, v. 34, n. 1, p. 92-6, 2010.

NOVAES, HMD Evaluation of programs, services and technologies in health . **Rev Saude Publica** , Sao Paulo, v. 34, n. 5, p. 547-559, 2000.

NOVAES, HMD; ELIAS, FTS Uso da valiaçao de tecnologia em saùde em procesos de anàlise para incorporaçao de tecnologia no Sistema Único de Saùde no Ministério da Saùde. **Cad Saùde Pùblica** , Rio de Janeiro, 29 Sup:57-516,2013.

NOBRE, Fernando et al. Controle da pressao arterial em pacientes sob tratamento anti-hypertensivo no Brasil: Controlar Brasil. **Arq Bras Cardiol** , v. 94, n. 5, p. 663-70, 2010.

OIGMAN, W. Métodos de avaliaçao da adesao ao tratamento anti-hypertensivo. **Rev Bras Hipertens** , Rio de Janeiro, v.13, n. 1, p. 30-34, Jan. 2006.

OLIVEIRA-FILHO, AD et al. The relationship between Morisky 's eight-item Therapeutic Adhesion Scale (MMAS-8) and blood pressure control . **Arq Bras Cardiol** , Sao Paulo, v.99, n.1, jul. 2012. Available< http://www.scielo.br/scielo.php?script=sci_arttext&pid =S0066-782X2012001000011&lng=pt&nrm=iso >. Accessed : 18 Jun 2013.

OLIVEIRA, RG *et al.* Accession of user interface and treatment hypertensive relationship with the family/Adesao do usuàrio hipertenso ao tratamento ea interface com o relacionamento familiar. **Revista de Enfermagem da UFPI** , v. 2, n. 4, p. 42-9, 2014.

OSTERBERG, L.; BLASCHKE, T. Adherence to medication. □**N Engl J Med** , v. 353, n. 5, p.487-497, 2005.

PANENI, F; COSTANTINO, S; COSENTINO, F. Insulin Resistance, Diabetes, and Cardiovascular Risk. **Current atherosclerosis reports** , v. 16, n. 7, p. 1-8, 2014.

PATEL , B.V. et *al* . Adherence with single-pill amlodipine/atorvastatin vs a two-pill regimen. **Vascular health and risk management** , v. 4, n. 3, p. 673, 2008.

PEDROSO, R. *et al.* A papel do programa national de acesso e da qualidade (PMAQ) no incentivo à educaçao permanente na atençao básica. In: **11th Congresso Internacional da Rede Unida** . 2014.

PERK, J. *et al* . bEuropean Association for Cardiovascular Prevention & Rehabilitation (EACPR) **Eur Heart J.** 2012;33(13):1635-701.

PIMENTA, AM *et al* . Açoes de prevençao de riscos e dinosados no setor suplementare de saùde. **Revista Mineira de Enfermagem** , v. 16, n. 4, p. 571-564, 2012.

PINHEIRO, J. C. **Trabalho feminino no Brasil: anàlise da evoluçâo da participaçâo da mulher no mercado de trabalho** (1950-2010). 2012.

PIRES, CG S,; MUSSI, FC Crenças em saùde para o controle da hipertensao arterial **. Cienc Saùde Coletiva** , Rio de Janeiro, v. 13, p. 2257-2267, dez. 2008.

PLADEVALL, M. *et al* . A multi-center cluster-randomized Trial of a multifactorial intervention to improve antihypertensive medication adherence and blood pressure control among patients at high cardiovascular risk (the COM99 study). **Circulation** , Dallas, v. 122, n. 12, p. 1183-1191, set. 2010. Available at: http://circ.ahajournals.org/content/122/12/1183 . Accessed: 02 Jun 2013.

POLIT, D. F.; BECK, CT; HUNGLER, BP **Fundamentos de pesquisa em enfermagem** : **methods, evaluation and utilization** . 5th ed. Porto Alegre: Artmed, 2004.

RAY, G. M.; NAWARSKAS, J.J .; ANDERSON, JR Blood pressure monitoring technique impacts hypertension treatment. **J Gen Intern Med** , Philadelphia, v. 27, n. 6, p. 623-9, Jun. 2012.

RIBEIRO, AG; **Adesao ao tratamento de portatores de HAS na atençao primárica à saùde** . Viçosa, 2011p. Dissertaçao (Mestrado em Ciência da Nutriçao).Departamento de nutriçao e saùde , Universidade Federal de Viçosa.

RIBEIRO, Amanda Gomes; COTTA, Rosângela Minardi Mitre; RIBEIRO, Sônia Machado Rocha. A promoçao da saùde ea prevençao integrada dos fáctores de risco para niños Cardiovasculares [The promotion of health and integrated prevention of risk factors for cardiovascular diseases]. **Ciênc Saùde Coletiva** , v. 17, n. 1, p. 7-17, 2012.

ROCHA, PQ *et al*. Cuidado e Tecnologia: Aproximaçao Atraves do Modelo de Cuidado. **Rev Bras Enferm,** Brasilia 2008 Jan-Feb;61(1):113-6.

ROHRBACHER, I. *et al* . "Orientaçoes de muñeca de estilo de vida em pacientes hypertensos." **AMRIGS Magazine** 58.1 (2014): 49-53.

SACKS, FM; *et al* . Effects on blood pressure of reduced dietary sodium and the Dietary Approaches to Stop Hypertension (DASH) diet. DASH-Sodium Collaborative. Research

Group. **N Engl J Med** 2001; 344: 3-10. S

SALOMAO, CB *et al.* Fatores associados à hypertensao arterial em usuarios de service de promotion à saùde. **Revista Mineira de Enfermagem** , v. 17, n. 1, p. 33-46, 2013.

SANTA HELENA *, et al* . **Adesao ao tratamento pharmacologico de usuarios com**

hypertensao arterial em unidades de saùde da familia em Blumenau, SC . Theses (Doutorado em Ciências) Universidade de Sao Paulo, Sao Paulo, 2007.

SANTA HELENA, E. T.; GERMAN, MIB; ELUF-NETO, José. Desenvolvimento e validaçao de questionàrio multidimensional para medir nao-adesao ao tratamento com medicamentos. **Revista de Saùde Pùblica** , v. 42, n. 4, p. 764-767, 2008.

SANTA HELENA *et al* . Fatores associados à nao-adesao ao tratamento com anti-hypertensivos em pessoas atendidas em unidades de saùde da familia. **I'm falling. Saùde Pùblica** , Rio de Janeiro, 26(12):2389-2398, Dec, 2010.

SARAFIDIS, PA; BAKRIS, George L. Resistant hypertension An overview of evaluation and treatment. **Journal of the American College of Cardiology** , v. 52, n. 22, p. 1749-1757, 2008.

SCHWARTZ, Bryan G.; REZKALLA, S.; KLONER, RA Cardiovascular effects of cocaine. **Circulation** , v. 122, n. 24, p. 2558-2569, 2010.

SANTOS, FP A; NERY, AA; MATUMOTO, S. A produçao do cuidado a usuarios com hypertensao arterial e as tecnologias em saùde. **Revista da Escola de Enfermagem da USP** , v. 47, n. 1, p. 107-114, 2013

SANTOS, HC M. *et al.* Metabolic syndrome and other risk factors for cardiovascular disease in the obese population . **rev. arm cardiol. (Impr.)** , v. 26, n. 6, p. 442-449, 2013.

SANTOS, Marcos Vinicius Ribeiro *et al.* Adesao ao tratamento anti-hypertensivo: conceitos, aferiçao e innovative strategies de approach; Compliance to treatment for hypertension: concepts, measurement, and innovative approach strategies. **rev. Shock. Arm. Clin. Med** , v. 11, n. 1, 2013.

SANTOS, ZMSA; SILVA. RM **Hypertensao arterial: modelo de educaçâo em saùde** para o selfcuidado. Fortaleza: UNIFOR, 2002.

SANTOS, ZMSA, FROTA, MA; NETHERLANDS, SDO; CRUZ, DM Adesao do cliente hypertenso ao tratamento - anâlise com arrondissement interdisciplinary. **Revista Texto e Contexto Enferm** 2005, v.14, n.3, p. 332-340.

SANTOS, ZMSA; LIMA, HP Açoes educativas na prevençao da hypertensao arterial em trabajoles. **Revista da Rede de Enfermagem do Nordeste-Rev Rene** , v. 9, n. 1, 2012.

SANTOS, ZMSA Multiprofessional and interdisciplinary service for hypertensive clients - doi: 10.5020/18061230.2004. p.86. **Revista Brasileira em Promoçao da Saùde** , v. 17, n. 2, p. 86-91, 2012.

SANTOS, ZMSA Adesao do cliente hypertenso ao tratamento: anâlise com arrondissement interdisciplinary. **Texto contexto** - enferm, Florianópolis, v. 14, n. 3, p. 332-340, Jul./Dec. 2005. Available at: < http://dx.doi.org/10.1590/S0104-07072005000300003 >. Accessed : 22 Jun 2013.

SILVA, LK Technological evaluation and cost-effectiveness analysis in health: the incorporation of technologies and the production of clinical guidelines for SUS. **Cienc Saude Coletiva** , Rio de Janeiro, v. 8, n. 2, feb. 2003.

SILVA, Mauriéli Escobar da *et al.* Elaboraçao de Material Explicativo sobre Alimentaçao Saudàvel e Cuidados Nutricionais nas Doenças Crônicas Non-Transmissiveis para Idosos de um Centro de Convivência. **Anais do Salao Internacional de Ensino, Pesquisa e Extensao** , v. 5, n. 3, 2013

SILVA, Silvio Fernandes yes. Organization of regional and integrated health care networks : challenges of the Unique Health System (Brazil). **Ciênc Saùde Coletiva,** v. 16, n. 6, p. 2753-62, 2011.

SILVA, Hudson P.; PETRAMALE, Clarice A.; ELIAS, Flavia TS. Advances and Challenges of the National Policy for the Management of Technologies in Health **. Revista de Saùde Pùblica** , v. 46, n. spe, p. 83-90, 2012.

SILVA, Wilson Rezende yes. The importance of planning. **Debates GVsaùde magazine** , n. 5, p. 8-9, 2014.

SOUZA, Ana Rita Araújo *et al.* A study on systemic arterial hypertension in the city of Campo Grande, MS. **Arquivos Brasileiros de Cardiology** , v. 88, n. 4, p. 441-446, 200

SOUZA, Elizabethe Cristina Fagundes de *et al* . Acesso e acolhimento na atençao básica: uma anâlise da perceptçao dos usuarios e professionales **. I'm falling. saùde pùblica** , v. 24, n. Sup 1, p. S100-S110, 2008.

SOUZA, Fernanda dos Reis. **Processo de construçâo dos nùcleos de apoio à saùde da familia (NASF) na atençao básica do estado do Cearà. 2013.**

SOUZA, MLP; GARNELO, L. "É muito dificultoso!": etnografía dos cuidados a pacientes com hipertensao e/ou diabetes na atençao básica, em Manaus, Amazonas, Brasil **. I'm falling. Saùde Pùblica** , Rio de Janeiro, 24 Sup. 1: S91-S99, 2008.

SOUSA P.; PEREIRA, MG, Intervençao na hypertensao arterial em doentes em cuidados de saùde primàrios. **PSYCHOLOGY, SAÙDE E DOENÇAS** , 2014, 15(1), 245-261

STESSEN, M. et al. The effect of coffee consumption on blood pressure and the development of hypertension: a systematic review and meta-analysis. **J Hypertens** 2012;30:2245-2254.

SUMAR, Norhan; FAUSTO, Marcia Cristina Rodrigues. Atençao Primària à Saùde: a construçao de um conceito ampliado. **JMPHC. Journal of Management and Primary**

Health Care , v. 5, n. 2, p. 202-212, 2014.

SVARSTAD, B. L. *et al.* The Brief Medication Questionnaire: a tool for screening patient adherence and barriers to adherence **. Patient Educ Couns** , v. 37, n. 2, p. 113-24, June 1999.

TAMBLYN, R., ABRAHAMOWICZ, M., DAUPHINEE, D., WENQHOFER, E., JACQUES, A.,

KLASS, D., HANLEY, JA, Influence of physicians' management, and communication ability on patient's persistence with antihypertensive medication. **Arch Intern Med** , Chicago, v.170, n. 12, 1064-1072, jun. 2010.

TRAVASSOS, C.; MARTINS, M. uma revisao sobre os conceitos de accesso e utilizaçao de serviços de saùde. **Cadernos de Saùde Pùblica** , Rio de Janeiro, n.20, Suppl.2, p.190-198, 2004.

TONELO,D,;PROVIDENCIA,R.;GONÇALVES,L.;Sindrome do Coraçao Pós-Feriado Revisto após 34 anos. **Arq Bras Cardiol** . 2013;101(2):183-189

VAN, O., HA, VERBERK, WJ, KROON, AA, *et al.* Effect of self-measurement of blood pressure on adherence to treatment in patients with mild-to-moderate hypertension. **J Hypertens** . 2010;28(3):622-7.48. Marquez-Contreras E, Martell-Claros N, Gil-Guillén V, et al

VASAN, RS, BEISER, A., SESHADRI, S., LARSON, MG, KANNEL, WB, D'AGOSTINO, RB, LEVY, D.,. Residual lifetime risk for developing hypertension in middle-aged women and men: The Framingham Heart Study. **Jama** , v. 287, n. 8, p. 1003-1010, 2002.

VELANDIA-ARIAS, A.; RIVERA-ALVAREZ, LN Agency for self-care and treatment adherence in persons with cardiovascular risk factors **. Rev Saude Publica** , Sao Paulo, v. 11, n. 4, p. 538-548, 2009.

V Diretriz Brasileira de Dislipidemias e Prevençao da Aterosclerose. Brazilian Society of Cardiology; 2013. **Arq Bras Cardiol** .2013;101 (4 Suppl.1) :1-22.

VI Diretrizes Brasileiras de Hipertensao Arterial 2010. **Arq Bras Cardiol** 2010;95 (1(Suppl.1):1-51).

VII Diretrizes Brasileiras de Hipertensao Arterial 2016. **Arq Bras Cardiol** 2016;107(3 Suppl.3):1-83.

VIANA, ALD et al. Health, development and technological innovation : the new approach and investigation perspective . **Lua Nova** , v. 83, p. 41-77, 2011.

VIDOT, DC; *et al* . Illicit drug use and cardiometabolic disease risk: an analysis of 2005-2008 National Health and Nutrition Examination Survey Data. **Int J Clin Pract** .2013 November ;67 (11)

WORLD HEALTH ORGANIZATION *et al.* 2003 World Health Organization (WHO)/International Society of Hypertension (ISH) statement on management of hypertension. **Journal of hypertension** , v. 21, n. 11, p. 1983-1992, 2003.

WORLD HEALTH ORGANIZATION (WHO). **Adherence to long-term therapies: evidence for action.** Geneva (Switzerland); 2003 WORLD HEALTH ORGANIZATION.

World Health Statistics , 2012. Geneva, Switzerland.

YUSUF, Salim *et al* . Effect of potentially modifiable risk factors associated with myocardial infarction in 52 countries (the INTERHEART study): case-control study. **The Lancet** , v. 364, n. 9438, pp. 937-952, 2004.

ZANELATTO, Neide A.; LARANJEIRA, Ronaldo. **O Tratamento da Dependência Quimica e as Terapias Cognitivo-Comportamentais: Um Guia Para Terapeutas** . Artmed, 2013.

ZELLER, A.; SCHROEDER, K.; PETERS, TJ Electronic pillboxes (MEMS) to assess the relationship between medication adherence and blood pressure control in primary care.

Scand J Prim Health Care , Oslo, v. 25, p. 202-207, 2007. Available at: http://www.ncbi.nlm.nih.gov/pubmed/179242 . Accessed: 07 Jun 2013

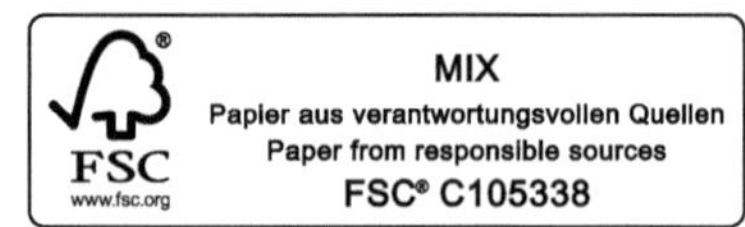

Printed by Books on Demand GmbH, Norderstedt / Germany